ESSENTIAL OPTICS REVIEW
FOR THE BOARDS

Second Edition. Revised and Expanded

Mark E. Wilkinson, OD
Clinical Professor of Ophthalmology
The University of Iowa
Carver College of Medicine

With a chapter on Contact Lens by
Ali Bukhamseen, OD, FAAO, FIACLE
Chief of Optometry Department
Saad Specialist Hospital
Al-Khobar, Saudi Arabia

Edited by Andrew P. Doan, MD, PhD

ESSENTIAL OPTICS REVIEW FOR THE BOARDS
second edition

By Mark E. Wilkinson, OD

Edited by Andrew P. Doan, MD, PhD

Published and distributed by F.E.P. International, Inc.
www.fepint.org
www.medrounds.org/optics-review/

Printed in the United States of America.

For information write F.E.P. International, Inc.
941 25th Avenue, #101
Coralville, IA 52241

ISBN 0-9769689-1-6

Line Drawings by Angie England
Copyediting and typesetting by Patricia Duffel
Cover Design by Daniel Hunt, www.sidekick-design.com

Advice and suggestions given in this book are not meant to replace professional medical care. The reader is advised to consult his or her physician before undertaking any diet or exercise regimen and in order to gain answers about or treatment for any medical problems. The authors and publisher have made every effort to ensure that drug selection and dosage set forth in this text are in accord with current recommendations and practice at the time of publication. However, because the practice of medicine may change with ongoing research, changes in government regulations, and developments in medicine, the reader is encouraged to read the package insert for each drug or medical device for any change in indications and dosage and for added warnings and precautions. This is particularly important when the recommended agent is a new or infrequently employed drug.

ABOUT THE AUTHOR

Mark E. Wilkinson, O.D. is co-author of *Protect Your Sight* and author of *Essential Optics Review for the Boards*. Dr. Wilkinson is a professor in the Department of Ophthalmology and Visual Sciences at the University of Iowa, which is one of the top ophthalmology teaching programs in the U.S. He is vice chair of the Executive Committee of the American Optometric Association Low Vision Rehabilitation Section. He has published extensively and spoken all over the globe concerning issues related to visual rehabilitation. He teaches optics to the ophthalmology residents at the University of Iowa and around the world.

To my wife Dana and our children, Lyndsey and Shaun

ESSENTIAL OPTICS REVIEW
FOR THE BOARDS

Table of Contents

iii

1. Light

a. Nature of Light

Light resembles sound in that it passes through a media; but unlike sound, it can also travel across a vacuum. This dual behavior of light, i.e. the ability to travel through a media as well as across a vacuum, has led to separate theories of its nature: wave theory and quantum theory.

Classically, light has been considered as a "stream of particles", a "stream of waves" or a "stream of quanta".

Physical Optics examines light as energy particles that are emitted by light sources and absorbed by other substances *(Wave or Quanta Theory of Light)*.
- *Wave Theory* helps to understand how light interacts with itself, different media and various surfaces. Wave theory allows us to understand the naturally occurring phenomena of interference, diffraction and polarization.
- Diffraction causes a decrease in normal visual acuity for apertures less than 2 mm (such as a very small pupil of the eye).

Geometric Optics deals with the formation of images by rays of light acted on by lenses, prisms and mirrors *(Particle Theory of Light)*.
- The concept of vergence is the unifying concept between wave theory and geometric optics.

Quantum Optics deals with the interaction of light and matter. It considers light as having both wave and particle (photon) characteristics. When light interacts with matter, photons are emitted or absorbed.
- Visible light is in the very narrow portion of the electromagnetic spectrum with wavelengths roughly between 400 and 800 nanometers ($380 - 760$nm or 4×10^{-6} m to 8×10^{-6} m). This portion of the electromagnetic spectrum represents approximately 1% of the sun's electromagnetic spectrum that ranges from 1×10^{-16} m to 1×10^{6} m.
- Yellow light is the standard wavelength for calibration. It holds mid position in the chromatic interval of the emmetropic eye and so is in best focus.
- A photon of wavelength 100 nm has 12.50 eV per photon. A photon of wavelength 193 nm has 6.4 eV per photon. This shows why shorter wavelengths of light (e.g. ultraviolet) have greater potential for photic damage, due to their higher energy level.

b. History of Light

- Newton, in 1665 stated that light was made of particles that moved in straight lines.
- One hundred years later, Kristian Huygens, a Dutch mathematician, suggested that the light was a wave form, after observing that a small amount of light was always bent onto the shadow behind an opaque object.
- Thomas Young proved the wave nature of light with a double slit defraction experiment.
- Einstein taught that the speed of light in a vacuum is always 186,000 miles per second regardless of the speed of the observer or the source. This was proven by the Michelson-Morely experiment. Einstein's work on light concluded that light really does act as a particle, but a particle that has wave properties.
- The Heisenberg principle rationalizes that when you try to measure something too precisely, the act of measurement itself, changes the thing being measured. This has led to light particles being called photons or quanta. Heisenberg suggested that quanta have wave properties.
  - o When light is considered as being composed of quanta, the results of all experiments and physical phenomenon can be predicted.
  - o A quanta of light's energy (E) is described by the equation $E = h\upsilon$, where υ is the frequency of the light wave and h is Planck's constant: 6.626×10^{-34} J/sec.
  - o Frequency and wavelength of light are related in the equation $c = wv$ where c = speed of light, v = frequency and w = wavelength. Therefore the constancy of the speed of light, c, guarantees a constant relationship between frequency and wavelength.

c. Movement of Light

- Movement of light by convention is from left to right. Positive numbers measure in the direction of light, negative measure against the direction of light. Therefore, a positive lens or waveform is converging and a negative lens or waveform is diverging.
- All naturally occurring wavefronts are diverging as they emerge from a source.
- As light rays approach infinity, they become parallel.
  - o Optical infinity is considered 20 feet (6 m) or greater.

2. Vergence

Vergence is defined as the reciprocal of the distance from a reference point (in meters) to the point of focus.

- Vergence is measured in diopters. (1 diopter = 1/1m = 100/100cm)
- The vergence of the light rays coming from an object is directly related to the distance from the object.

In Figure 1, the divergence of rays of light emanating from point O is,

at A, 1/–0.25 = –4.00D;

at B, 1/–0.50 = –2.00D;

at C, 1/–1 = –1.00D;

at D, 1/–2 = –0.50D and

at E, 1/–3 = –0.33D.

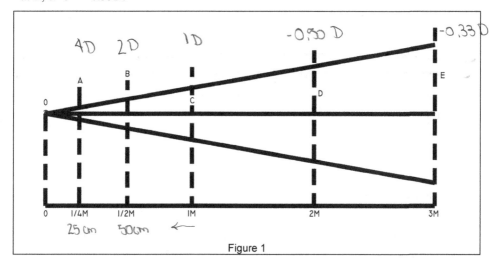

Figure 1

In Figure 2, the convergence of the rays of light, converging to the point I is, at A, 1/4 = +0.25D; at B, 1/3 = +0.33D; at C, 1/2 = +0.50D, at D, 1/1 = +1.00D and at E, 1/0.5 = +2.00D

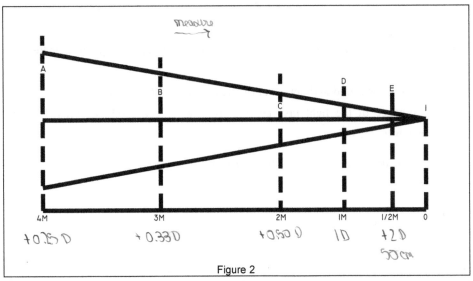

Figure 2

By convention, divergence is given in minus (–) vergence power and convergence is given in plus (+) vergence power.

- Convergent wavefronts are not found spontaneously in nature. They are the result of an alteration of a planar or divergent wavefront by a refractive or reflective medium.
- An object (O) is defined as a point or extended source that the pencil/beam of light comes from.
- The object's distance from the object to the point of reference is designated as u.
- The object's vergence (U) is the distance from the object to the point of reference. U = 100/u (cm)
- The image (I) is defined as a point or extended source that the pencil/beam of rays go to.
- The image distance is measured from the point of reference to the image and is defined as v.
- The image's vergence (V) is the distance from the image to the point of reference.
- V = 100/v (cm)
- When defining an optical system, it is conventional to set the incoming rays as object rays, the outgoing rays as image rays, and light travels from left to right.

Definition. Diopter: a unit of accommodative amplitude; it describes the vergence of a waveform and describes the vergence at a specific distance from the source; and it is also defined as the power of the lens. A diopter is the reciprocal of the distance in meters.

3. Lens Systems

Objects and Images for Lens Systems *(Figure 3)*

- Real objects have diverging rays and are on the same side as the incoming object rays.
- Virtual objects are not naturally occurring and have converging rays.
- Real images have a focal point that can be focused on a screen and therefore are on the same side as the outgoing image rays.
- Virtual images cannot be focused on a screen and are always on the left side of the lens system.
- A virtual object may also have a virtual image.
- When light rays are about to cross, they are considered to have positive (+) vergence (convergence) and when they are receding from their crossing point, they are said to have negative (–) vergence (divergence).
- Rays that cross at the focal point of the lens are considered to have an infinite amount of vergence. Therefore rays that are parallel (have no crossing point), have a vergence of zero.
- Converging lenses have real/inverted images that are on the opposite side of the lens from the object.
- Diverging lenses create virtual/erect images that are on the same side as the object.

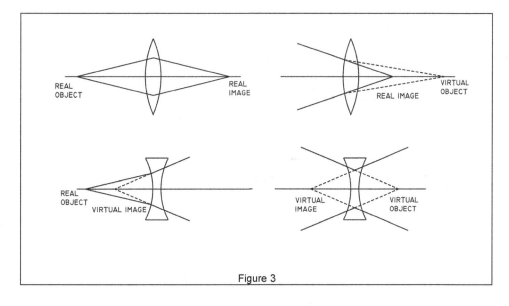

Figure 3

4. Simple Lens Formula

$U + D = V$ or 100/u (cm) + D = 100/v (cm)

Where: U = vergence of object at the lens   u = object position = 100/U (cm)

               D = lens power

               V = vergence of image rays   v = image position = 100/V (cm)

Vergence: The reciprocal of the distance from a reference point. U = 100/u, where u is measured in centimeters or U = 40/u where u is measured in inches.

**NOTE: Light travels from left to right unless otherwise stated.

**NOTE: Light never comes out of the eyes.

Question: If parallel light rays strike a +4.00D lens, where will the image be? (Figure 4)

Answer: Parallel light has no vergence. Therefore, using the equation $U + D = V$
U = vergence of object at the lens = 0.00D
D = lens power = +4.00D

Vergence of image rays = V = 0.00D + (+4.00D) = +4.00D.
Converting to centimeters, 100cm/+4.00D = +25 cm to the right of the lens.

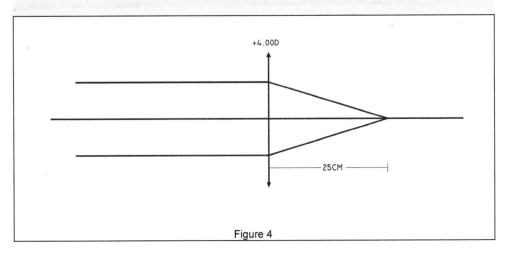

Figure 4

Question: An object is placed 25 cm in front of a refracting surface of power +10.0D. (Figure 5)

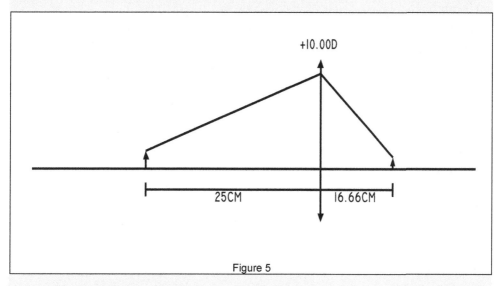

+10.00D

25CM   16.66CM

Figure 5

1. What is the image vergence?

Use the equation U + D = V
U = object vergence = –4.00D
D = lens power = +10.00D
V = image vergence= –4.00D +(+10.00D) = +6.00D

2. Where is the image placed?

To find the location of the image, the image vergence (V) is converted into cm.
Use the equation, v = image position = 100/V where V = +6.00D
v = image position = 100/+6 = +16.66 cm to the right of the lens.

3. Is the image real?

Yes, because its position is positive and to the right of the lens.

Question: An object is located 25 cm in front of a +5.00D lens.

1.   What is the vergence of the incident rays?

Use the following equation to calculate the object vergence: U = 100/u

Where u = object location in cm

U = object vergence = 100/–25 = –4.00D

$$\frac{1}{-.25} = -4.00\,D$$

o   .15m   +5.00

2.   What is the refracting vergence?

$V = F + U$

$V = 5 \cdot 4$

$V = 1$

Use the equation U + D = V where

U = object vergence = –4.00D

D = lens power = +5.00D

V = refracting vergence of the image = –4.00D + (+5.00D) = +1.00D

3.   Where is the image located?

Use the equation, v = image position = 100/V where V = +1.00D

v = image position = 100/+1 = +100 cm to the right of the lens.

$$V = \frac{1}{l} \qquad 1 = \frac{1}{l} \qquad l = 1m$$

4.   Is the image real or virtual?

Real   found to right which is real image space

Question: Define a plus lens

Answer: Plus lenses always add vergence; define a focal point; and converge image rays to produce a real image of an object at infinity to the right of a plus lens.

Question: Define a minus lens

Answer: A minus lens always reduces vergence; defines a focal point; and diverges image rays to produce a virtual image of an object at infinity to the left of the minus lens.

Question: What is the focal length of a plus lens whose image is 20 cm behind the lens for an object that is 50 cm in front of the lens? (Figure 6)

Answer: First, determine the lens power by using the equation U + D = V where

     u = object distance = –50cm

     v = image distance = +20cm

     U = object vergence = 100/u = 100/–50 = –2.00D

     D = lens power

     V = image vergence = 100/v = 100/20 = +5.00D

$$\frac{1}{-.5} + P = \frac{1}{.2}$$
$$-2 + P = 5$$
$$P = 7.00D$$
$$7 = \frac{1}{f} = +.143\,m$$

Lens power = D = V – U = +5.00D – (–2.00D) = +7.00D

Therefore, the focal length (f) of the lens, in cm, is 100/D, f = 100/+7.00D = +14.29cm.

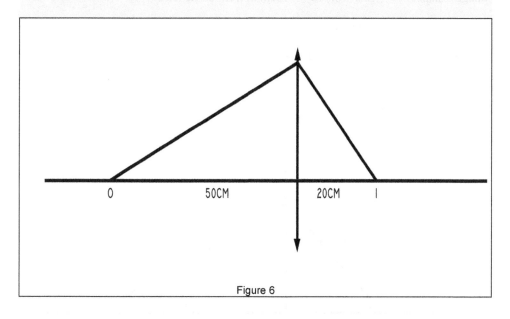

0   50CM   20CM   I

Figure 6

Question: An object is imaged 20cm behind a –15.00D lens. (Figure 7)

1. Is the object real or virtual?

Virtual, because it is behind the lens.

2. Where will the image be focused?

Use the equation U + D = V where

u = object distance = +20cm

U = object vergence = 100/u = 100/+20 = +5.00D

D = lens power = –15.00D

V = image vergence = +5.00D + (–15.00D) = –10.00D

image distance = v = 100/–10.00D = –10cm in front of the lens.

3. Is the image real or virtual?

Virtual, because it is in front of the lens.

$+5 = u$

$-15 = P$

$-10 = V$

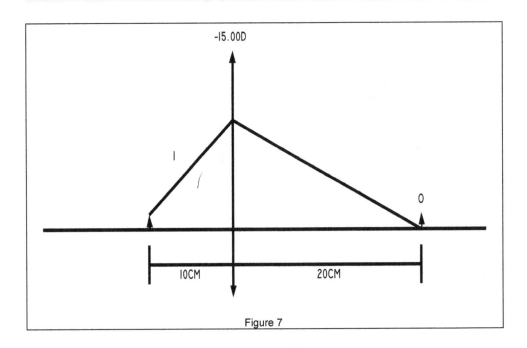

Figure 7

5. Depth of Focus

Depth of focus describes the image location range where the image is clear when focused by an optical system. Outside this range, the image will be significantly blurry. However, within this few millimeter range, the image appears quite sharp.

6. Depth of Field

Depth of field is the same principle for objects as the depth of focus is for images. When an optical system such as the camera is focused on an object, nearby objects are also in focus, inside the camera's depth of field. Objects outside of the depth of field will be out of focus.

7. Multiple Lens Systems

When working with a multiple lens system, it is essential to first calculate the position of the image formed by the first lens. Only after locating the first image is it possible to calculate the vergence of light as it reaches the second lens. This is the method by which any number of lenses can be analyzed. Always remember to locate the image formed by the first lens and use it as the object for the second lens to calculate the vergence of light as it reaches the second lens. Repeat the process for each subsequent lens.

Question: Where will the image be formed for an object placed 50cm in front of a +4.00D lens that is separated from a –2.00D lens by 25cm. (Figure 8) $-2+4 = 2$ 50 cm

Answer: First, determine the vergence of the image of the object after it passes through the first lens (+4.00D).
Use the equation $U_1 + D_1 = V_1$ for the first image, where
u_1 = object distance = –50cm
U_1 = object vergence = $100/u_1$ = 100/–50 = –2.00D
D_1 = Lens 1 power = +4.00D
V_1 = image vergence = $U_1 + D_1$ = –2.00D + (+4.00D) = +2.00D
Therefore, Image 1 focuses at v_1 = $100/V_1$ = 100/+2.00D = +50cm behind Lens 1.
Now, Image 1 becomes Object 2 ($I_1 = O_2$).

At Lens 2 (–2.00D), Object 2 is located +50cm behind Lens 1 and +25cm behind Lens 2 because Lens 2 is 25cm from Lens 1.

Object 2 has a vergence of U_2 = $100/u_2$ = 100/+25 = +4.00D

11

Using the formula $U_2 + D_2 = V_2$ where

U_2 = Object 2 vergence = +4.00D

D_2 = Lens 2 power = –2.00D

V_2 = Image 2 vergence = $U_2 + D_2$ = +4.00 + (–2.00) = +2.00D. Therefore, Image 2 focuses at $v_2 = 100/V_2 = 100/+2.00D$ = +50cm behind Lens 2.

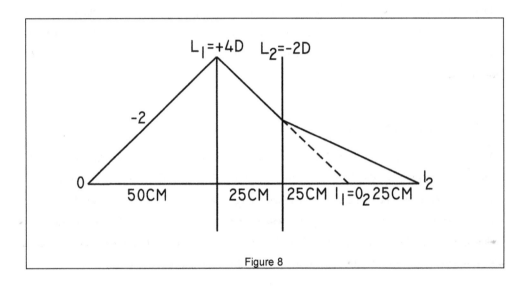

Figure 8

Question: Consider an object 10cm in front of a +5.00D lens in air. Light strikes the lens with a vergence of $100/u = 100/-10 = -10.00D$. (Figure 9)

The image has a vergence of $V = U + D = -10.00D + (+5.00D) = -5.00D$. In this case, light emerges with a negative vergence, which means the light is still diverging after crossing the lens. No real image is produced. In this case, we have a real object and a virtual image. Now suppose that a +6.00D thin lens is placed 5 cm behind the first lens.

1. Will an object be formed?
2. If so, what are its characteristics?

Image 1 becomes Object 2 and has a vergence of $-5.00D$. As the light crosses the 5cm to the second lens, its vergence changes. In order to determine the vergence at the second lens, it is necessary to find the location of the image formed by the first lens. If the first lens does not form a real image, it has a virtual image. As light leaves the first lens, it has a vergence of $-5.00D$. The same vergence would be produced by an object 20cm away if the first lens were not present. So, as light leaves the second lens, it appears to be coming from an object 20cm to the left of the first lens and 25cm away from the second lens. Therefore, the vergence at the second lens is $U_2 = 100/u_2 = 100/-25cm = -4.00D$. When light leaves the second lens, it has a vergence of $V_2 = U_2 + D_2 = -4.00D + (+6.00D) = +2.00D$ forming a real image 50cm ($v = 100/V = 100/+2.00D$) to the right of the second lens.

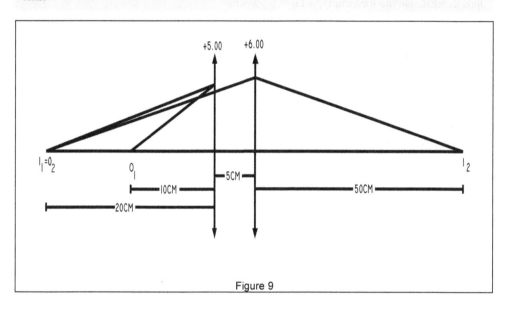

Figure 9

Question: A +2.00D and a –3.00D lens are separated by 30cm. The final image is 20cm behind the second lens (–3.00D). (Figure 10) Where is the object located?

Answer: In this case we need to work backwards. Using the formula $U_2 + D_2 = V_2$ where

v_2 = Image 2 distance = +20cm
U_2 = Object 2 vergence
D_2 = Lens 2 power = –3.00D
V_2 = Image 2 vergence = $100/v_2$ = 100/+20cm = +5.00D

$U_2 = V_2 – D_2$ = +5.00D – (–3.00D) = +8.00D.
Therefore, the location of Image 1/Object 2 is v_1=100/V_1 =100/+8.00 = +12.5cm right of lens 2. Next, use the formula $U_1 + D_1 = V_1$ where

v_1 = Image 1 distance from Lens 1 = +30 cm + 12.5cm = +42.5cm
U_1 = Object 1 vergence
D_1 = Lens 1 power = +2.00D
V_1 = Image 1 vergence = $100/v_1$ = 100/+42.5 = +2.35

$U_1 = V_1 – D_1$ = +2.35 – (+2.00D) = +0.35D. Therefore, object 1 is located at u_1 = 100/U_1 = 100/+0.35D = +285.71cm to the right of the first lens.

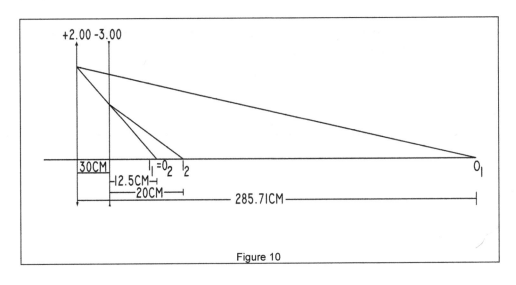

Figure 10

8. Lens Effectivity

Lens effectivity is the change in vergence of light that occurs at different points along its path. This is related to vertex distance.

Formula: $F_{new} = F_{current}/(1-dF_{current})$ where F is in Diopters and d is in meters.

When providing a "distance correction", the principle focal point F_2 of the correcting lens must coincide with the far point of the eye. The lens power depends on its location in front of the eye. The closer to the eye the lens is mounted, the shorter is its focal length in the case of hyperopia, and the longer its focal length in the case of myopia. Because of this, plus power has to be added in both cases. Therefore, myopes need less minus and hyperopes need more plus when going from spectacles to contact lenses.

Remember **CAP – Closer Add Plus**.

For spectacles, pushing a minus lens closer to the eyes increases the effective power of the lens (more –). Moving a plus lens away from the eyes increases the effective power of the lens (more +).

Question: A +12.00 diopter lens mounted 12mm in front of the cornea would require what contact lens power?

Answer: $F_{new} = F_{current}/(1-dF_{current}) = +12.00/(1-0.012(+12.00)) = +14.02D$

Question: For a myopic eye that can be corrected with a –12.00 diopter lens mounted 12 mm in front of the cornea would require what contact lens power?

Answer: $F_{new} = F_{current}/(1-dF_{current}) = -12.00/(1-0.012(-12.00)) = -10.49D$

Question: An object is placed 0.3m in front of a +5.00D lens. (Figure 11) What lens power could be used 0.2m from the image to achieve the same effectivity?

Answer: First, we need to –know where the image will be focused.

Using the equation U + D = V where
u = object distance = –30cm
U = object vergence = 100/u = 100/–30cm = –3.33D
D = lens power = +5.00D
V = image vergence = U + D = –3.33D + (+5.00D) = +1.66D
v = image distance = 100/V = 100/+1.66D = 60cm to the right of the lens. Therefore the image is 30cm + 60cm = 90cm from the object and the new lens will be 90cm – 20cm = 70cm from the object.

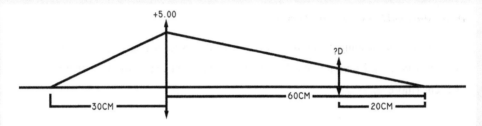

Figure 11

For the new lens, use the equation U + D = V where

u = –70cm
U = object vergence = 100/–70 = –1.43D
v = image distance = +20cm
V = image vergence = 100/+20cm = +5.00D
D = new lens power = V – U = +5.00D – (–1.43D) = + 6.43D (the lens power needed to achieve the same effectivity).

9. Focal Points

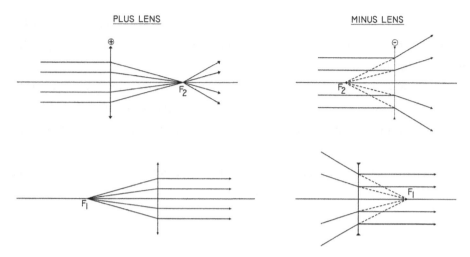

Figure 12

- The primary focal point (F₁) of a lens is also called the Object-Space Focus.
    - For a plus lens, this is the point from which light must originate to emerge parallel from the lens. Thus, the image is at infinity.
    - For a minus lens, this is the point towards which the incident light must be directed in order for the image rays to emerge parallel.
- The primary focal length, (f₁), is the distance from the optical surface to the primary focal point (F₁).
- Secondary focal point (F₂) of a lens is also called the Image-Space Focus.
    - For a plus lens, this is the point where parallel rays from a distant point object are rejoined to form an image at that point. When parallel rays enter the optical surface, they will focus at the secondary focal point.
    - For a minus lens, this is the point from which diverging rays seem to come from, after a parallel bundle of rays are refracted by a negative lens.
- The secondary focal length, (f₂), is the distance from the optical surface to the secondary focal point (F₂).
- For a plus (+)/convergent lens, the secondary focal point is to the right of the lens.
- For a minus (–)/divergent lens, the secondary focal point is to the left of the lens.

10. Ray Tracing – Lenses

When performing ray tracing, there are three rays that follow simple known paths before and after their refraction by the lens. Use two of the three construction rays to find the image. (figures 13 A & B)

1. Draw a line from the object to the lens, parallel with the direction of light. At the lens, draw the line through the secondary focal point of the lens.

2. Draw a line from the object, through the center of the lens (no deviation at the lens).

3. Draw a line from the object to F_1 and then to the lens. At the lens, draw the line parallel with the direction of light.

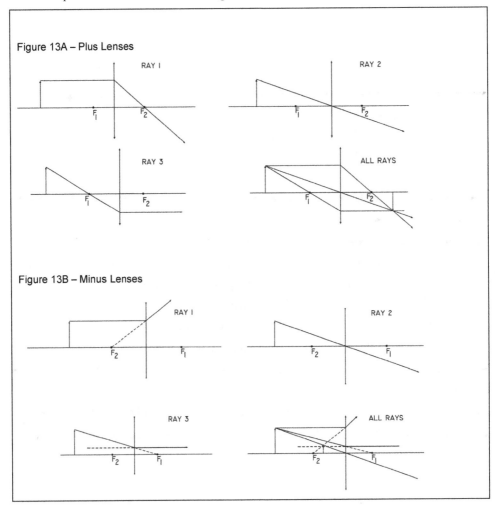

Figure 13A – Plus Lenses

Figure 13B – Minus Lenses

Where the lines cross is where the image will be. By doing this, you can estimate the approximate location of the image, tell whether the image is erect or inverted as well as real or virtual.

Figures 14 show the construction of images produced by a plus lens:
a)   Object farther from the lens than F_1 , image is real
b)   Object lies in F_1 plane, the image therefore is at infinity
c)   Object closer to lens than F_1 , image is virtual
d)   Object at infinity, image at F_2.
e)   Object lies to the right of the lens, (a virtual image projected by another optical system), image is real.

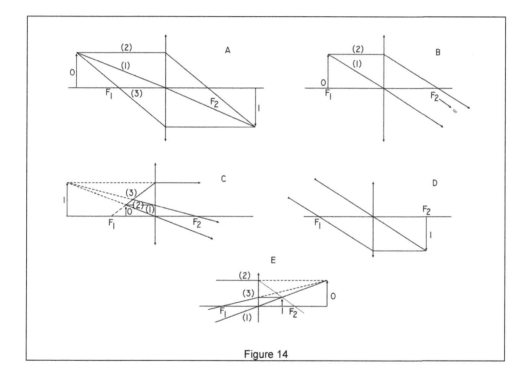

Figure 14

Figure 15 shows the construction of images produced by a minus lens:

a)   Object real, image virtual

b)   Object at infinity, image at F_2 plane

c)   Virtual object in F_1 plane, image at infinity

d)   Virtual object closer to lens than F_1, image real

e)   Virtual object farther than F_1, image virtual

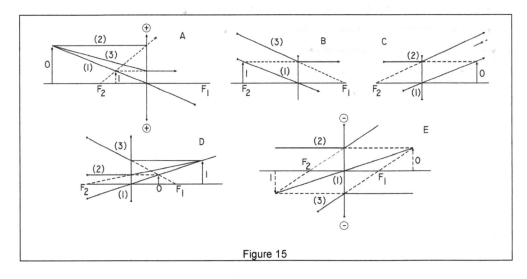

Figure 15

11. Optical Media and Indices of Refraction

A medium is any material that transmits light. Light travels at different speeds in different media. Light travels faster in a vacuum and slower through any material. A medium's refractive index (n) = speed of light in a vacuum (c)/speed of light in a particular medium (v). Refractive indices are always equal to or greater than 1.0. The index tells us how much light has slowed down when entering a refractive media. Denser media have higher n values; rarer media have smaller n values.

- Vacuum = 1.00
- Air is assumed to be 1.00
- Water, aqueous, vitreous = 1.33

- Averaged corneal refractive index used for keratometry = 1.3375
- Cornea = 1.37
- Crystalline lens = 1.42
- Plastic (CR-39) = 1.49
- Crown glass = 1.52
- Polycarbonate (higher index than glass or plastic) = 1.59
- High index glasses = 1.6/1.7/1.8
- Titanium glass is now available with an index of 1.806. However, it is 2 ½ times heavier than CR-39.

With higher index lenses, chromatic aberration becomes a factor (chromatic aberration is discussed in Section 20). Although higher index glass lenses are thinner, they have a higher specific gravity and so are considerably heavier than plastic or crown glass. Polycarbonate lenses continue to be the lens of choice, because of its greater safety and lighter weight.

As light goes from a vacuum to a medium, the light waves slow down slightly. The denser the medium, the slower they move.

Object vergence $V = n/u$

Image vergence $V' = n'/u'$

Where: n = index of refraction for where the light is coming from

           n' = index of refraction for where the light is going to

           u = object distance

           u' = image distance

Question: If light of wavelength 460nm encounters the interface of a new medium with an index refraction of 1.24, find the reduced wavelength of the new medium.

Answer: When light encounters a denser medium, the frequency remains constant. Therefore, the speed of light is reduced compared to that inside a vacuum, and thus, the wavelength must be reduced to maintain $c = wv$. Vergence is inversely related to wavelength and is thus, increased. The light rays may emerge with the same frequency, wavelength, or be reflected or refracted. To calculate the wavelength in the new medium:

$w_m = w/n = 460/1.24 = 371$ nm

12. Snell's Law of Refraction

If light hits the surface of a media at less than a 90° angle, the angle formed between the line representing the path of light and a line that is perpendicular to the surface (the so called normal line), is called the angle of incidence. The line representing the light that emerges on the other side of the interface, measured from the normal line, is called the angle of refraction. (Figure 16)

n sin i = n' sin r where: i = angle of incidence as measured from the normal

r = angle refracted as measured from the normal

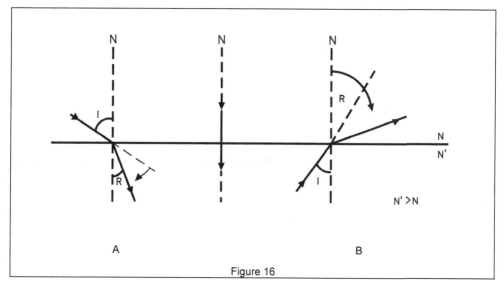

Figure 16

When light enters a denser media at an angle, it slows down so that the path becomes a bit more perpendicular. Therefore light assumes a more nearly perpendicular path when passing from a less dense, into a denser medium, but assumes a less perpendicular path when passing from a denser medium into a less dense one.

- When moving from rarer to denser medium, light is bent towards the normal. (Figure 16 A)
- When moving from a denser to a rarer medium, light is bent away from normal. (Figure 16 B)

Question: Light leaves a medium of n = 1.55 at an angle of 30° to the normal, how much does the angle change in air?

Answer: Using n sin i = n' sin r where

n = index of refraction of the medium where light is coming from = 1.55

i = angle of incidence = 30°

n' = index of refraction of air = 1

r = angle of refraction = (n sin i)/n' = (1.55 sin 30°)/1 = 50.81°. Therefore the angle would change 50.81° – 30° = 20.81°.

Question: Define refraction of light.

Answer: Refraction is the bending of light between media and is a function of the incident angle. This is based on Snell's Law and is not dependent on the speed of light. Snell's Law is the relationship between the incident and refracted angles of the light ray. It has no bearing on the Law of Reflection.

Question: What happens to light as it travels from a less dense to a denser medium?

Answer: It is refracted towards the normal. If it travels from a more dense to a less dense medium, it is refracted away from the normal.

Question: What happens to a beam of light, perpendicular to the interface between two media, as it emerges from the more a dense medium?

Answer: It is transmitted at a higher speed.

13. Apparent Thickness Formula

Apparent Thickness Formula: n/u = n'/u'

Where: n = index of refraction for where the light is coming from

n' = index of refraction for where the light is going to

u = object distance

u' = image distance

Question: A butterfly is embedded 10cm deep in a piece of CR-39 (n = 1.498) lens material. How far into the lens material does the butterfly appear to be?

Answer: Using the formula n/u = n'/u', 1.498/10cm = 1/u', u' = 10cm/1.498 = 6.68cm.

**NOTE: Light leaves the object of regard, not the eye. In this case, although we are looking into the block of plastic at the butterfly, light is coming from the butterfly. For this reason, n = 1.498.

Question: If a fisherman is going to spear a fish that is 50cm below the surface of the water, which he sees at an angle of 40° from the surface of the water, where should he aim to spear the fish? (Figure 17)

Answer: The image that is viewed, as 40° from the surface of the water will be 50° from the normal (a line perpendicular with the surface of the water).

Using the formula n sin i = n' sin r; 1.33 sin i = 1 sin 50°; i = 35.17°
Using the formula n/u = n'/u'; 1.33/50 cm = 1/u'; u' = 50cm/1.33 = 37.59cm

Therefore, the fisherman should aim behind and below the fish because light from the fish is passing from a more dense to a less dense medium and will be refracted away from the normal. The fisherman sees a virtual image ahead of and above the actual fish.

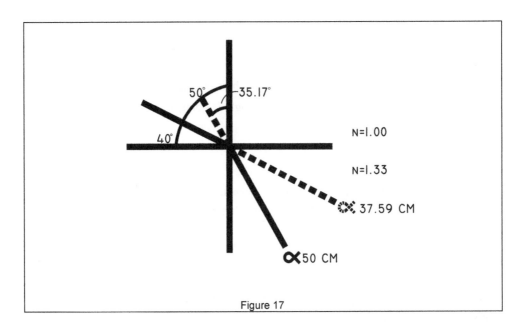

Figure 17

Reflection and refraction of smooth surfaces

When light enters a medium, it may be: reflected off the surface, refracted (bending of light due to a change in velocity when it hits the medium) or absorbed (where it is changed into a different type of energy).

14. Law of Reflection and Critical Angle

The *Law of Reflection* A = a' where A = angle of incidence and a' equals the angle of reflection. The angle of incidence and the angle of reflection are both measured from a normal to the surface. The normal is at 90° to the surface the light is hitting. (figure 18)

The *Critical Angle* occurs when going from a *denser to a rarer* medium. There is a point where a' = 90° and all light is therefore internally reflected. The angle of incidence (a) that produces this condition is termed the Critical Angle (CA). Total internal reflection occurs when the angle exceeds CA. *As n increases, CA decreases.* The angle can be determined using Snell's law as follows:

n sin i_c = n' sin 90°   where: i_c = the critical angle and the refracted angle is 90°,

$$\sin i_c = n'/n \times 1$$

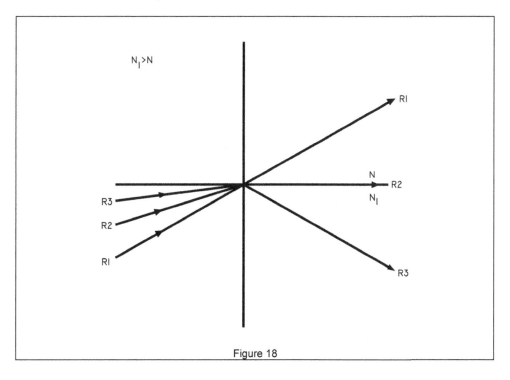

Figure 18

As the refractive index increases, the critical angle decreases. The refractive index of blue light is greater than the refractive index of red light. For this reason, blue light has a smaller critical angle than red light.

Question: If light is passing through a prism and hits the second surface at the critical angle for the blue wavelength, red light will be:

a)   totally internally reflected
b)   will be refracted
c)   this system is not subject to chromatic dispersion

Answer: b, because the critical angle of red light is greater than that for blue light

Question: What is the critical angle when going from water to air?

Answer: Use Snell's law $n (\sin i_c) = n' (\sin 90°)$

i_c = the critical angle
refracted angle is $90°$
n = index of refraction for water = 1.33
n' = index of refraction for air = 1.00
$(\sin i_c) = n'/n \times 1 = 1/1.33 = 48.75°$

Question: What is the critical angle when going from a CR-39 (n = 1.4988) lens to air.

Answer: Use Snell's law $n (\sin i_c) = n' (\sin r)$

i_c = the critical angle
n = index of refraction of CR-39 = 1.4988
n' = index of refraction of air = 1.00
r = $90°$
$\sin i_c = n'/n \times \sin 90° = 1/1.498 \times 1 = 41.88°$

Question: What types of ophthalmic instruments are the applications of the critical angle the basis for?

Answer: Fiberoptics, gonioscopy, reflecting prisms, and Goldmann lens funduscopy. It is not related to retinoscopy.

15. Mirrors

- The focal length of a curved mirror is always ½ its radius of curvature ($f = r/2$)
  - o f = focal length of the mirror in meters
  - o   The reflecting power of a mirror in diopters $D_M = 1/f$ (m)
  - o r = radius of curvature of the mirror in meters.
  - o   For mirrors or reflecting surfaces: $U + 2/r_m = V$, (r_m is in meters) or $U + 1/f = V$
- If the mirror is convergent or plus, the focal point is to the left of the mirror.
- If the focal point is to the right of the mirror, the mirror is divergent or minus.
- Convex mirrors form virtual images on the opposite side from the object.
- Concave mirrors form real images on the same side as the object.
- A plus (concave) mirror adds positive vergence, while a minus (convex) mirror adds minus vergence.
- Convex mirrors add negative vergence like minus lenses.
- Concave mirrors add positive vergences like plus lenses.
- Plane mirrors add no vergence.
- The field of view of a plane mirror is 2 times its size.
  - o   Holding a hand mirror farther away from the face does not enlarge the field of view.
  - o   You need approximately a 1/2 length mirror to see your entire self.

When the object is located closer to a converging lens or a converging mirror than its focal distance, the image will be virtual and erect, not real and inverted. These are the principles applied to magnifying glasses used to read small print and a concave mirror, used as a shaving mirror.

Question: (Figure 19) Consider a concave mirror whose radius of curvature is 50cm. Therefore, the focal length of the mirror is $f = r/2 = 0.5/2 = 0.25$m, and the reflecting power of the mirror is $1/f = 1/0.25 = +4.00$D.

a)   If an object lies 1m in front of the mirror, where is the image vergence?

Answer:
Use the equation $U + D = V$ where
$u = -1$m $= -100$ cm
U = object vergence = $100/u = 100/(-100) = -1.00$D
D = reflecting power of the mirror = $+4.00$D
V = image vergence = $U + D = -1.00$D $+ (+4.00$D$) = +3.00$D
Therefore the image is real and lies 33cm in front of the mirror.

b) If an object point is 50cm in front of the mirror, which coincides with C – the center of curvature, the image vergence (–2 + 4 = +2) also coincides with C.

c) If an object point coincides with F, the focal point of the mirror, the image vergence (–4 + 4 = 0) is at infinity.

d) If an object point lies 20cm in front of the mirror, the image point (–5 + 4 = –1) is virtual (reflected rays are divergent) and lies 1m in back of the mirror.

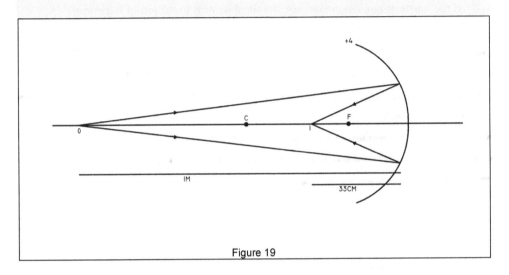

Figure 19

Question: (Figure 20) Consider a convex mirror whose radius of curvature is 40cm. Therefore, the focal length of the mirror is f = – (r/2) = –0.4/2 = –0.20m, and the reflecting power of the mirror is 1/f = 1/–0.20 = –5.00D.

If an object lies 1m in front of the mirror, what is the image vergence?

Answer:
Use the equation U + D = V where
u = –1m = –100 cm
U = object vergence = 100/u = 100/(–100) = –1.00D
D = reflecting power of the mirror = –5.00D
V = image vergence = U + D = –1.00D + (–5.00D) = –6.00D
Therefore the image is virtual and lies 16.67cm behind the mirror.

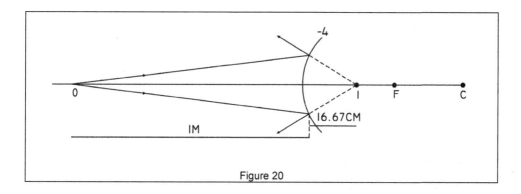

Figure 20

Question: For a cornea with a radius of curvature of 8mm, what is the reflective power of the cornea?

Answer:
The cornea is a convex mirror, and its reflective power is negative. The focal length of the cornea is f = – (r/2) = –(0.008/2) = –0.004m, and the reflecting power of the cornea is 1/f = 1/–0.004 = –250D.

16. Ray Tracings – Mirrors

(Figures 21 & 22)

When doing ray tracings, there are three rays that follow simple known paths before and after their refraction by the mirror, just as there were with lenses. Use two of the three construction rays to find the image.

1. Draw a line from the object to the mirror, parallel with the direction of light. At the lens, draw the line through the primary focal point of the mirror.

2. Draw a line from the object, through the center of curvature of the mirror, then to the mirror.

3. Draw a line from the object to F and then to the mirror. At the mirror, draw the line back parallel to the axis of the mirror.

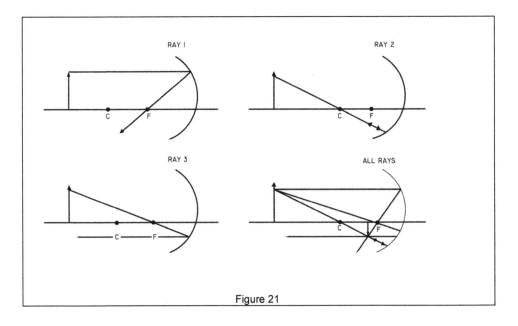

Figure 21

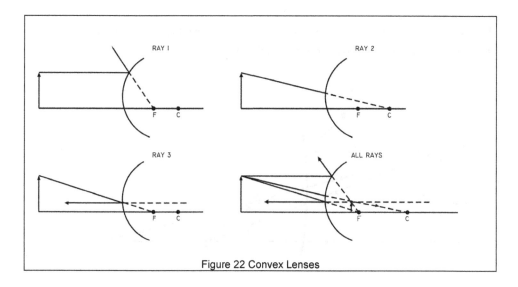

Figure 22 Convex Lenses

Where the lines cross is where the image will be formed. By doing this, you can estimate the approximate location of the image, tell whether the image is erect or inverted as well as real or virtual.

Figure 23 shows the construction of mirror images produced by a concave mirror:

a) Object farther from mirror than C, image real and inverted
b) Object at C, image also at C, real and inverted
c) Object at F, image at infinity
d) Object closer to mirror than F, image virtual and erect

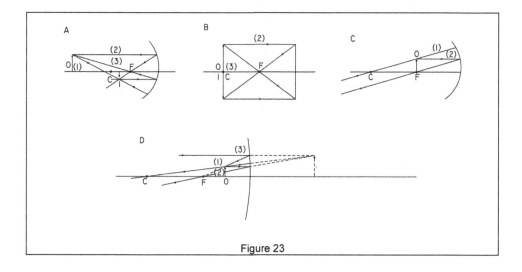

Figure 23

Figure 24 shows the construction of mirror images produced by a convex mirror:

- Object real, image virtual, erect and minified.

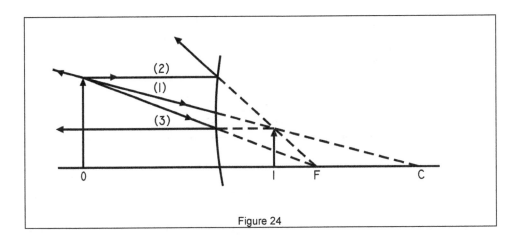

Figure 24

Plane Mirror: (Figure 25)

This mirror has a power of zero. Therefore U = V and m = +1. This indicates that any real object has a virtual erect image of the same size and any virtual object has a real, erect image of the same size. The virtual image of a real object will be located as far behind the mirror as the real image is in front of the mirror.

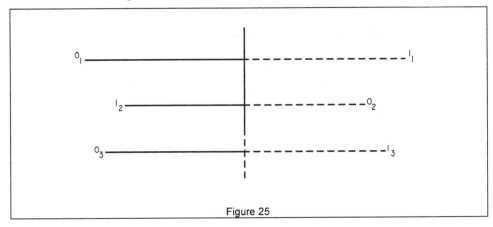

Figure 25

Question: An object is placed 1m to the left of a concave mirror with a radius of curvature of 20cm. Where will the image be focused? Will the image be real or virtual; magnified or minified; erect or inverted? Additionally, do a line drawing to show these results. (Figure 26)

Answer:
The focal length of the mirror (f) = r/2 = 0.2/2 = 0.10m.
The power of the mirror (D_m) = 1/f = 1/0.10 = +10.00D.

The position of the image is:
u = object distance = –1m
U = object vergence = 1/u = 1/(–1) = –1.00D
D_m = reflecting power of the mirror = +10.00D
V = image vergence = U + D_m = –1.00D + (+10.00D) = +9.00D

Image position is v = 100/V = 100/+9.00 = +11.11cm.
Magnification = U/V = –1.00D/+9.00D = –0.11.
Therefore, the image will be real, inverted and minified.

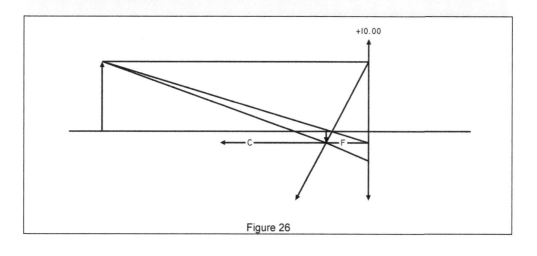

+10.00

Figure 26

Question: (Figure 27) An object is placed 0.5m to the left of a cornea with a radius of curvature of 10mm. Where will the image be focused? Will the image be real or virtual; magnified or minified; erect or inverted? Additionally, do a line drawing to show these results.

Answer:

The focal length of the cornea (f) = $-$ (r/2) = $-0.01/2$ = -0.005m.

The reflective power of this cornea is (D_m) = 1/f = 1/-0.005 = -200.00D.

U = object vergence = 1/u = 1/(-0.5) = -2.00

V = image vergence = U + D_m = -2.00D + ($-$v200.00D) = -202D

Image position = v = 1000/V = 1000/-202 = -4.95mm.

Magnification = M = U/V = $-2/-202$ = 0.0099.

Therefore, the image will be virtual, erect and minified.

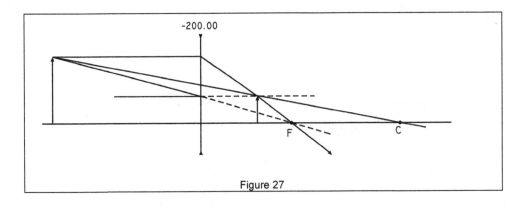

Figure 27

17. Prisms

Prisms are defined as a transparent medium that is bound by two plane sides that are inclined at an angle to each other. Prisms are used to deviate light, but do not change the vergence and for this reason, they do not focus light. With prisms, light is bent towards the base. The image of an object formed by a prism is a virtual image. The image will appear displaced towards the apex of the prism.

A *Prism Diopter* ($^\Delta$) (See Figure 28) is defined as a deviation of 1 cm at 1 meter. For angles under 45° (or 100$^\Delta$), each degree (°) of angular deviation equals approximately 2$^\Delta$ *(Approximation Formula)*.

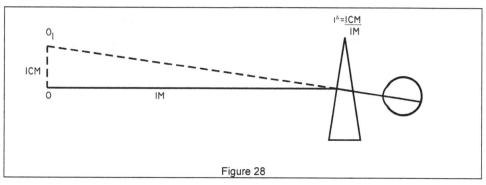

Figure 28

Question: A 6 PD prism will displace a ray of light how far at 1/3m?

Answer: A 6PD prism will deviate light 6cm at 1m. Therefore at 1/3m x 6PD = 2cm.

Question: What is the power of a prism that displaces an object 10cm at a distance of 50cm?

Answer: 10/50 = x/100 = 20PD.

18. Prentice's Rule

Prentice's Rule determines how much deviation you get by looking off center of a lens. There is no prismatic power at the optical center of the lens. Deviation in prism diopters (PD) = h (cm) x F where F = power of the lens and h = distance from the optical center of the lens.

**NOTE: a plus lens is really 2 prisms stacked base to base and a minus lens is 2 prisms stacked apex to apex.

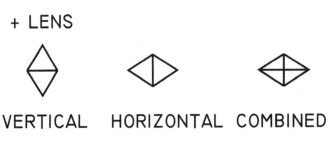

+ LENS

VERTICAL   HORIZONTAL   COMBINED

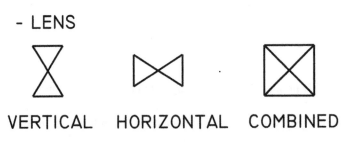

- LENS

VERTICAL   HORIZONTAL   COMBINED

$3 \times 5 = 1.5^\triangle BU$

$.5 BD$

$2.0^\triangle BU\ OD$

Question: A patient wearing glasses with these lenses, OD: +3.00, OS: −1.00, complains of vertical diplopia when reading. Both eyes are reading 5 mm down from the optical center. How much total prism is induced in this reading position?

Answer:

Use Prentice's rule: PD = hF where h = distance from optical center in centimeters and F = power of the lens.

Therefore, in the right eye, 0.5cm x 3.00D = 1.5 prism diopters base up (inferior segment of a plus lens), and in the left eye, 0.5cm x 1.00D = 0.5 prism diopters base down (inferior segment of a minus lens). Total induced vertical prism is 2.0 prism diopters.

Question: What is the induced prism for an individual wearing +5.00D OU, when reading at the usual reading position of 2mm in and 8mm down from the optical center of his lenses?

Answer:

Use Prentice's rule: $PD = hF$

Therefore, vertically $5.00D \times 0.8 = 4PD$ BU per eye (inferior segment of a plus lens) and horizontally $5.00D \times 0.2 = 1PD$ BO per eye (nasal segment of a plus lens)

Spectacles provide a prismatic effect in viewing strabismic deviations. A plus lens will decrease the measured deviation, whether it is esotropia, exotropia or hyper/hypotropia. A minus lens increases the measured deviation, whether it is esotropia, exotropia or hyper/hypotropia. The true deviation is changed by approximately 2.5% per diopter.

For example, an exotrope of 40^{Δ} wearing –10.00D spherical glasses will measure 2.5 (10) = 25% more exotropia, for a total measured deviation of 50^{Δ} XT.

NOTE: the 3M mnemonic - **Minus **M**easures **M**ore

Convergence (in prism diopters) required for an ametrope to bi-fixate a near object is equal to the dioptric distance from the object to the center of rotation of the eyes, multiplied by the subject's intra-pupillary distance in centimeters.

Convergence $(^{\Delta})$ = 100/working distance (cm) x Pupillary Distance (cm)

Question: What is the convergence required by an individual with a 60mm intra-pupillary distance when viewing an object at 40cm?

Answer:
Convergence $(^{\Delta})$ = 100/working distance (cm) x Pupillary Distance (cm)
100/working distance (cm) = 100/40cm = 2.50D
Pupillary Distance (cm) = 6cm
Convergence $(^{\Delta})$ = 2.50D x 6 = 15 prism diopters of convergence

19. Lenses

a. Surface type

– Spherical - power and radius is the same in all meridians

– Aspheric - radius changes from the center to the outside (becomes less curved usually)

– Cylindrical- different powers in different meridians

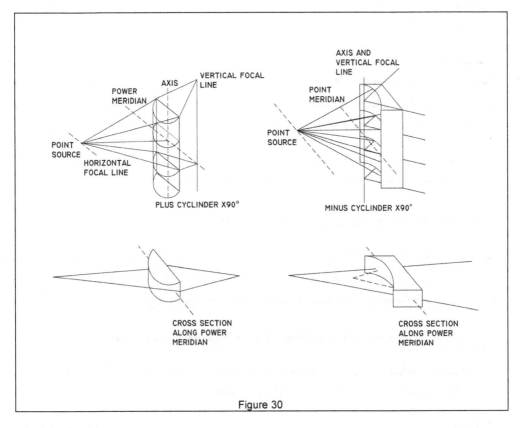

Figure 30

b. Cylinder Optics

The power meridian is always 90 degrees away from the axis. Therefore, if the axis is 45 degrees, the power meridian is at 135 degrees. (Figure 30)

Example: Plano + 5.00 x 45 = +5.00 @ 135 and Plano @ 45

- A cylinder is specified by its axis
- The power of a cylinder in its axis meridian is zero.
- Maximum power is 90 degrees away from the axis. This is known as the power meridian.
- The image formed by the power meridian is a focal line parallel to the axis.

- Example: Plano + 5.00 x 045 will have a focal line at 45 degrees.
- There is no line focus image formed by the axis meridian, because the axis meridian has no power.

c. Astigmatism Types

minus   150 , 030

With the rule astigmatism is corrected with a ~~plus~~ cylinder lens between 60 and 120 degrees.

minus   060   Ro

Against the rule astigmatism is corrected with a ~~plus~~ cylinder between ~~150~~ and ~~30~~ degrees.

Therefore, **oblique astigmatism** is from 31 to 59 and 121 to 149 degrees.

Irregular astigmatism occurs when by retinoscopy or keratometry, the principal meridians of the cornea, as a whole, are not perpendicular to one another. Although all eyes have at least a small amount of irregular astigmatism, this term is clinically used only for grossly irregular corneas such as those occurring with keratoconus or corneal scars. Cylindrical spectacle lenses can do little to improve vision in these cases, and so for best optical correction, rigid contact lenses are needed.

d. Astigmatism of Oblique Incidence

Tilting a spherical lens produces astigmatism. Tilting a plus lens induces plus cylinder with its axis in the axis of tilt. Tilting a minus lens induces minus cylinder with its axis in the axis of tilt. Therefore, if a lens is tilted along its horizontal axis, the increased plus or minus astigmatism will occur along axis 180. A small amount of additional sphere of the same sign is induced as well.

e. The Interval or Conoid of Sturm

The interval is a conical image space bound by the two focal lines of a spherocylinder lens. At the center of the Conoid of Sturm is the *Circle of Least Confusion. (Figure 31)* The Circle of Least Confusion is the dioptric midpoint of a cylindrical lens and is defined as the *spherical equivalent* of the cylindrical lens. This is where the horizontal and vertical dimensions of the blurred image are approximately equal. The goal of a spherical refractive correction is to choose a lens that places the Circle of Least Confusion on the retina. The smaller the Interval of Sturm, the smaller is the blur circle (Circle of Least Confusion).

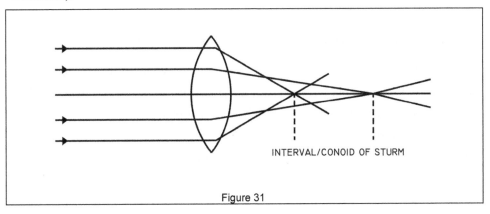

INTERVAL/CONOID OF STURM

Figure 31

f. Spherical Equivalent

Dioptric midpoint of a sphero-cylindrical lens. ½ cylinder power + sphere power. This is also known as the Circle of Least Confusion.

When one wishes to utilize only partial correction of the astigmatism, it is still desirable to keep the circle of least confusion on the retina. This is why we use the spherical equivalent formula to maintain the circle of least confusion on the retina.

g. Power Transposition: converting plus to minus cylinder and vice versa

To convert plus to minus cylinder and vice versa, add sphere power to cylinder power = new sphere power, change sign of cylinder power, change axis by 90 degrees.

Examples: +2.50 +3.50 x 95 = +6.00 – 3.50 x 005

                            –2.75 – 2.00 x 010 = –4.75 + 2.00 x 100

h. Base Curves of Lenses

- The base curve is used to designate the lens form.
- The base curve varies not only for different ranges of power but also for the same ranges of powers among different lens manufacturers.
- The following definitions are standard for lenses (exceptions can be found):
  - For single vision spherical lenses it is the weaker of the two curves. The base curve will be the back or concave side of a plus lens and the front or convex side of a minus lens.
  - For astigmatic single vision lenses, it is the lesser (weaker/flatter) of the two curves on the side in which the cylinder is ground. For plus cylinder form lenses, the cylinder is ground on the front surface of the lens while for minus cylinder form lenses, the cylinder is ground on the back surface of the lens.
  - Because almost all lenses are designed in a minus cylinder form, manufacturers identify their lenses in terms of the front curve.
  - For multifocal lenses, the base curve is on the spherical side containing the reading segment.

20. Aberrations

a. Chromatic (color) Aberrations

is the change in light direction in materials with different refractive index due to the different wavelengths of light. A simple plus lens will bend blue light rays more than red rays, leading to the optical aberration known as chromatic aberration. The blue rays come to focus closer to the lens than the red rays. Chromatic aberration occurs strongly in the human eye; with almost 3.00D difference in the focus of the far ends the visible spectrum. This is the basis of the red-green test used for refinement of the sphere power in clinical refraction.

b. Chromatic dispersion

is caused because each wavelength of light has its own index of refraction. Shorter wavelengths (blue) deviate the most in materials with higher index of refraction.

Aberration can be modified by
- Changing the shape of the lens
- Changing the refractive index of the lens
- Changing the aperture size (results in fewer marginal rays)
- Changing the position of the aperture

In general, it is not possible to eliminate all aberration at once. Minimize one may worsen the other; therefore we need to prioritize and minimize the most irritating aberrations.
- Aberrations are all object/image distance dependent.

c. Monochromatic Aberration

is caused by non-paraxial rays of light. Monochromatic aberrations include spherical aberration, coma, oblique astigmatism, curvature of field and distortion.

i. Spherical aberration

is shape dependent. Spherical aberration normally increases as you move towards the peripheral portion of the lens. This is because the deviating power of the lens increases towards the periphery of the lens (Prentice Rule). To minimize spherical aberration, a biconvex lens is used. Aspheric lenses, lenses where the radius of curvature gets flatter in the periphery (have less power at the edge of the lens) also help minimize aberrations. The cornea is an aspheric surface that gradually flattens towards the periphery.

ii. Aperture size:

The larger the aperture, the more spherical aberration from marginal rays occurs. Increasing pupil diameter causes greater spherical aberration. This is due to off axis points or extended objects that result in light rays passing through the marginal surface of the lens. This results in the lens not focusing the image at the same point due to para-axial rays. The difference in angles causes the aberration. The pupil of the eye corrects spherical aberration and coma.

iii. Coma

is an off axis spherical aberration. Peripheral rays produce coma. The image is a series of circles that form a comet shape. This is primarily a problem for large aperture optical systems and can be ignored in spectacles because of the limited affect of the pupil. If we increase the aperture size, we have more coma. Shorter objects have less coma. Objects off axis have more coma. Lens shape will minimize spherical aberration, but not totally eliminate coma. When the aperture is closer to the lens, greater coma occurs.

iv. Aplanatic system

is free of spherical aberration and coma.

v. Curvature of field

is corrected by the curvature of the retina. Curvature of field is an advantageous aberration in the human eye because it produces a curved image on the retina, as opposed to a flat image.

vi. Distortion

Distortion (Figure 32) is another aberration of thick lenses. It concerns the distortion of straight edges of square objects. There are two types of distortion resulting from lateral magnification of the image that results in a lateral displacement of the image.

- *Barrel distortion* - where the rays in the center are more magnified than the rays further off axis. This is due to minification of the corners of a square object, more then the sides, from minus lenses.

- *Pincushion* - where the central rays are less magnified than the rays off axis. This is due to magnification of the corners of a square object, more then the sides, from plus lenses.

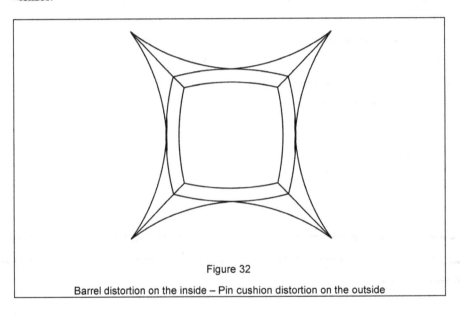

Figure 32

Barrel distortion on the inside – Pin cushion distortion on the outside

21. Schematic Eye

A schematic eye (Figure 33) helps to conceptualize the optical properties of the human eye. The reduced schematic eye treats the eye as if it were a single refracting element consisting of an ideal spherical surface separating two media of refractive indices of 1.00 and 1.33. The reduced schematic eye assumes an eye power at the corneal surface of +60.00D (actual power of the Gullstrand's schematic eye is +58.60D). The anterior focal point is approximately 17mm (1/–60 = –16.67mm in front of the cornea) and the eye is 22.6mm in length with the nodal point 5.6mm behind the cornea.

The nodal point is the point in the eye where light entering or leaving the eye and passing through the nodal point, is undeviated. This allows similar triangles to be used to determine the retinal image size of an object in space. For example, to determine the retinal image size of a Snellen letter (viewed at 6 meters), the following formula would be used: Retinal image height/Snellen letter height = 17mm/6000mm

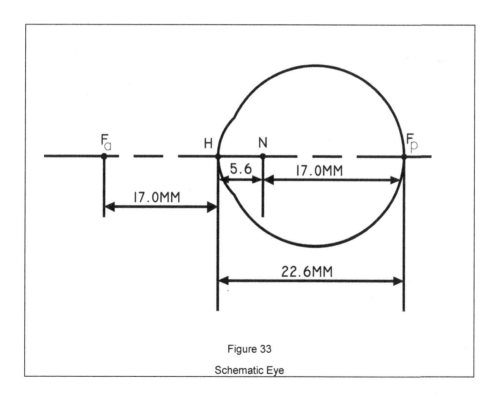

Figure 33
Schematic Eye

Question: Assume a disc diameter of 1.7 mm. What is the diameter of the blind spot when plotted on a tangent screen 2 meters from the eye?

Answer: Using similar triangles, $1.7/17 = X / 2,000$. Rearranging $X = 1.7/17$ x $2,000 = 200$ mm or 20 cm. In general, you can use the formula: object height/retinal image height = distance from the point of reference/17 mm. 17mm is the distance from the internal focal point of the eye to the retina.

22. Refractive/Axial Myopia and Hyperopia

Refractive Myopia: occurs when the power of the eye exceeds 60D and the length of the eye is 22.6mm. This is due to steeper corneal curvatures or higher lenticular powers.

Axial Myopia: occurs when the power of the eye is 60D but the eye is longer than 22.6mm. Every millimeter of axial elongation causes approximately 3D of myopia.

Refractive Hyperopia: occurs when the power of the eye is less than 60D and the length of the eye is 22.6mm.

Axial Hyperopia: occurs when the power of the eye is 60D but the eye is shorter than 22.6mm.

23. Knapp's Law

One problem in treating refractive errors is that the corrective lens usually changes the size of the retinal image. Many individuals can tolerate this change in image size. Problems can arise with differences in image size between the two eyes, because of asymmetric refractive errors. According to Knapp's Law, the retinal image size will not be different between the two eyes, no matter what amount of axial ametropia exist, when the spectacle lens is placed at the eye's anterior focal point. The front focal point of the eye is about 17 mm in front of the cornea (see schematic eye information). Preventing this from being strictly applied in clinical practice is the fact that ametropia is almost never purely axial, and a vertex distance of 16-17 mm for a spectacle correction is impractical. Most people prefer to wear their spectacles 10-14 mm in front of the cornea. Additionally, the retina in the myopic eye of a unilaterally high myope is stretched, which increases the separation of photoreceptors. This results in the effective magnification not being exactly what would be expected.

24. Far Point of the Eye

The far point of the eye is the object point imaged by the eye onto the retina in an unaccommodated eye. If a corrective lens is used to correct for myopia, the lens has its secondary focal point coincident with the far point of the eye.

- The far point of the emmetropic eye is at infinity.
- Myopia exists if, without accommodation, a point at infinity is imaged in front of the retina (in the vitreous). The stimulus on the retina is therefore not a point, but a blur circle. Moving the object closer to the myopic eye, until the image is a point focus on the retina, establishes the far point of the eye.
- Hyperopia exists, if without accommodation, an object point at infinity is imaged neither in the vitreous nor on the retina, but theoretically, behind it.

25. Accommodation

Accommodation is the mechanism by which the eye changes its refractive power by altering the shape of its crystalline lens. During accommodation, the ciliary muscle contracts allowing the zonular fibers to relax. This relaxation causes the equatorial edge of the lens to move away from the sclera during accommodation resulting in increased lens convexity (roundness). This increase in roundness primarily occurs on the front surface of the lens.

a. The *Amplitude of Accommodation,*
also known as the accommodative response, is the maximum increase in diopter power obtainable by an eye. The amplitude of accommodation is measured monocularly.

b. The *Range of Accommodation*
denotes the linear distance (expressed in centimeters or meters) over which the accommodative power allows an individual to maintain clear vision. The range lies between the near point of accommodation and the far point of accommodation. This is considered the most useful clinical measurement of accommodation. It helps answer the question as to whether an individual's accommodative range comfortably encompasses his visual needs.

Clinically, accommodative ranges are measured from the anterior corneal surface (reference position). Optically, for the purist, that reference should be the primary principle plane of the eye, 1.4 mm behind the anterior corneal surface.

c. Resting Level of Accommodation:
In the absence of visual stimuli, the eye assumes an accommodative posture approximately 1D inside the far point, at the so-called "dark focus". This phenomenon helps explain "night" myopia and "empty field" myopia. Activation of the sympathetic nervous system is apparently involved in driving the accommodative state from the resting level to the far point in ordinary seeing.

d. Measuring Accommodation:
Tests of accommodation are performed monocularly.

When measuring the accommodative amplitude, it is assumed that you are testing an emmetropia, or someone who is corrected with spectacles, so that their far point is at infinity.

Target size, target illumination, and speed of target approach will affect the measurement of the amplitude of accommodation. The push up method works well for emmetropes, or fully corrected ametropes.

i. Near point of accommodation "Push Up Test"
For this test, use relatively small letters (0.4M or 0.5M) to help better control accommodation. Slowly move these letters closer to the eye until they become blurry. Measure the distance the letters became blurry. This is the near point of accommodation.

ii. Prince Rule
A scaled accommodative ruler is used. Normally it is done with +3.00D sphere over the distance correction. A standard reading card is used and moved slowly towards and away from the individual to locate both the near and far points as in the push up method.

Question: An emmetrope views the reading card through a +3.00 diopter lens. She finds that as the card is moved towards her, the print that was blurred when held at the far end of the prince scale (50 cm) becomes clear at 33 cm (3.00D) and remains clear until it reaches 10 cm (10D). What is her accommodative amplitude?

Answer: Accommodative amplitude then is 7 diopters, 10D – 3D.

iii. Spherical Lens Test
Spherical lenses are used in this test. The individual focuses on a stationery target while plus or minus lenses are used to measure the accommodative amplitude. A reading card is put at a convenient distance, say 40 cm, and the individual fixates on threshold size type (0.5M). Plus lenses are added until the print is blurred and then minus spheres are gradually added until the print blurs again. The difference is the accommodative amplitude.

Always test for accommodate relaxation with plus lenses before performing accommodative stimulation with minus lenses. This is because some individuals cannot adequately relax accommodation after exerting a maximum accommodative effort.

During the act of accommodation, there is a thickening of the lens and a decrease in its diameter (vertically and horizontally), with at the same time, a protrusion forward of the center and a relative flattening of the periphery, the whole process being accomplished by an axial movement of the lens substance which is evident, particularly in the central regions (Duke-Elder, 1938)

Question: What is the interval of clear vision for an uncorrected 5.00D myope with 10D of accommodative amplitude?

   Answer: Far point = 100/5 = 20cm
                    Near point = 100/(5 + 10) = 6.67cm
                    Interval of clear vision = 6.67cm to 20cm

Question: What is the interval of clear vision for an uncorrected 2.00D hyperope with 4.00D of accommodative amplitude?

   Answer: Far point is 50 cm behind the eye
                    With +2.00D of accommodation, the far point is at infinity
                    Near point = 100/(4–2) = 50cm
                    Interval of clear vision is 50cm to infinity

Question: What is the relative effect of spectacles versus contact lenses on convergence for a myope? For a hyperope?

Answer: When wearing contact lenses, the convergence requirement is the same as that of an emmetrope, because the lenses rotate with the eye and the line of sight remains relatively well directed through the center of the lenses. When an ametrope wearing spectacle lenses centered for his distance pupillary distance fixates a near object, the amount of convergence required is not only a function of his intrapupillary distance and the distance of the object, but will also be a function of the refracting power of the spectacle lenses. As a myope converges to bi-fixate a near object, his line of sight departs from the center of his spectacle lenses and encounters increasing amounts of base in prismatic effect. The spectacle wearing hyperope encounters base out prismatic effect, as he converges to bi-fixate a near object. Thus, to bi-fixate a given object at a distance less than infinity, the bespectacled myope converges less than the emmetrope or the contact lens wearer, while the hyperope wearing spectacles converges more than the emmetrope or the contact lens wearer. Therefore, the myope who discards his spectacle lenses in favor of contact lenses, must converge more to bi-fixate a given near object, while the hyperope will converge less under the same conditions.

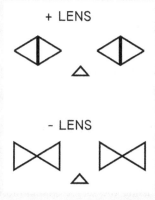

26. Near Point of the Eye

The near point of the eye is found when the uncorrected refractive error of the eye is added to the accommodative ability of the eye. If the amplitude of accommodation is 10D, the near point is 10cm in front of the eye (specifically, 10cm in front of the vertex of the cornea which is used as a convenient reference point).

When a myope is fit with contact lenses, they may experience asthenopia, or "focusing" difficulties when doing close work. The symptoms generally subside as the individual adapts to the greater accommodative stimulus. However, this can be a more of a problem for the myope who is approaching presbyopia. This is because the myope, when viewing a near object, will accommodate more when his ametropia is corrected with contact lenses than when it is corrected with spectacle lenses.

For the hyperope who is approaching presbyopia, they will experience less difficulty when reading with a full contact lens correction than with the equivalent spectacle lens correction. This is because the hyperope, under the same conditions, will accommodate less with contact lenses than with spectacle lenses.

The effect is greatest with high refractive errors. For example, a spectacle-corrected myope may be able to read without bifocal glasses, but require reading glasses with contact lenses. Conversely, a hyperope may be able to forego reading glasses with contact lenses, but need bifocal glasses when wearing spectacles.

The change in lens position from the spectacle plane to the corneal plane is primarily responsible for the change in the stimulus to accommodation.

Question: In general, when using the direct ophthalmoscope, which patient provides the larger image of the retina, the hyperope or myope?

Answer: Myopes will have a larger image, hyperopes smaller. This is related to the total power of the eye.

Question: Where is the secondary focal point for an uncorrected myope found?

Answer: The secondary focal point for a myopic eye is anterior to the retina.

Question: Where is the secondary focal point for an uncorrected hyperope found?

Answer: The secondary focal point for a hyperopic eye is behind the retina.

Question: Where is the far point for an uncorrected myopic eye found?

Answer: The far point is between the cornea and infinity.

Question: Where is the far point for an uncorrected hyperopic eye found?

Answer: The far point is beyond infinity or behind the eye.

27. Magnification

Traditionally, three types of magnification are discussed: relative distance magnification, relative size magnification, and angular magnification.

a. Relative Distance Magnification

The easiest way to magnify an object is to bring the object closer to the eye. By moving the object of regard closer to the eye, the size of the image on the retina is enlarged. Children with visual impairments do this naturally. Adults will require reading glasses to have the object in focus.

- Relative Distance Magnification = r/d where r = reference or original working distance and d = new working distance
- Example
    - Original working distance = 40cm
    - New working distance = 10cm
    - Relative Distance Magnification (RDM) = 40/10 = 4x

With reading glasses, as the lens power increases, the working distance decreases. The reading glasses do not magnify by their power alone when worn in the spectacle plane. Magnification occurs because the lens strength requires the individual using them to hold things closer to have the object in focus.

b. Relative Size Magnification

Relative size magnification enlarges the object while maintaining the same working distance, for instance, as observed with large print.

- Relative Size Magnification = S2/S1 where S1 = original size and S2 = the new size
- Example
    - Original size = 1M
    - New size = 2M
    - Relative Size Magnification (RSM) = 2/1 = 2x

c. Angular Magnification

Angular magnification (Figure 34) occurs when the object is not changed in position or size, but has an optical system interposed between the object and the eye to make the object appear larger.

Examples: Telescopes and hand magnifiers

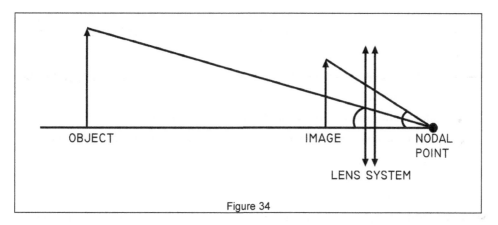

OBJECT   IMAGE   NODAL
                                                                  POINT

LENS SYSTEM

Figure 34

This optical system produces a virtual image smaller than the original object but much closer to the eye. The image has a larger angular subtense than the original object; therefore, the objects appear larger when seen through this optical system even though the virtual image is smaller than the object.

Angular magnification is the ratio of the angular subtense of the image produced by a device divided by the angular subtense of the original object. Angular magnification takes into account not only the size of an image, but also its distance from the observer.

d. Magnification Basics

- Perceived size is proportional to the size of the object's image on the retina.
- Retinal image size is proportional to the object's angular subtense.
- Angular subtense is directly proportional to the object size and inversely proportional to the object's distance from the observer.

Magnification looks at the ratio of object size (Y) to the image size (Y') or the ratio of the angular subtense of the image viewed with the optical system to the angular subtense of the object viewed without the optical system.

- Plus (+) indicates the image is upright
- Minus (–) indicates the image is inverted

- When the image is smaller than the object, magnification is numerically between 0-1.
- If the absolute number is greater than 1, the image is larger.
- If the absolute number is equal to 1, it is the same size.
  - A magnification of −4 implies that the image is inverted and 4x larger than the object
  - A magnification of 0.2 implies that the image is erect and 1/5 the size of the object.
- If the object and image are on the same side of the lens, the image is erect, if not, the image is inverted.
- Generally, if the image is located farther from the lens than the object is, the image is larger than the object, if the image is closer to the lens than the object; the image is smaller than the object.

e. Transverse/Linear Magnification

The ratio of the image size to the object size or image vergence to object vergence is called transverse or linear magnification. (Figure 35) $M_T = I/O = U/V = v/u$

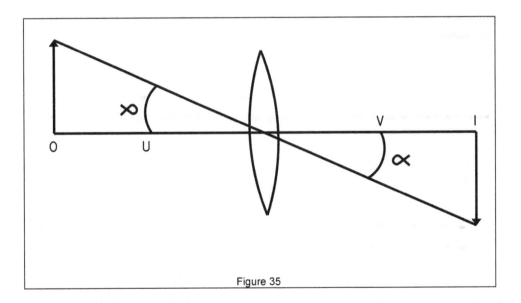

Figure 35

Question: An object is placed 20cm in front of a +10.00 diopter lens. What will the resultant linear magnification be?

Answer: −1

Explanation: In order to calculate linear magnification for a single lens system, one must know only the object distance and the image distance and/or the object vergence and the image vergence.

The formula is *Magnification = image distance (v)/object distance (u) = U/V*.

If the object distance is 20cm, the rays incident on the lens have a vergence of 100/–20 = –5.00D. After refraction, through the +10.00 diopter lens, the rays have a vergence of –5.00 + (+10.00D) = +5.00D. Therefore, a real image is formed 100/+5.00D = +20cm behind the lens.

As it turns out, the object distance of 20cm and the image distance of 20cm, are equal, so the magnification is –1. Also the object vergence is –5.00D and the image vergence is +5.00D giving a magnification of –5.00/+5.00 of –1, indicating the image is inverted.

Question: Consider an optical system consisting of two lenses in air. (Figure 36) The first lens is +5.00D, the second lens is +8.00D and they are separated by 45 cm. If an object is 1 meter in front of the first lens, where is the final image and what is the transverse magnification?

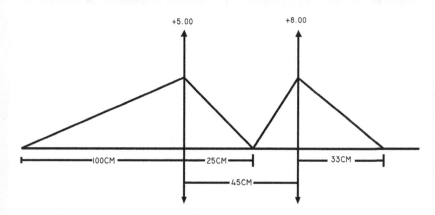

Figure 36

Answer: To analyze a combination of lenses, we must look at each lens individually. The thin lens equation (U + D = V = 1/–1 + (+5.00) = –1 +5 = +4.00D and 100/+4.00 = +25cm) shows that the first lens produces an image 25cm behind itself, with the magnification (M = U/V = –1/+4 = –0.25). Light converges to the image and then diverges again. The image formed by the first lens becomes an object for the second lens. The image is 20 cm in front of the second lens, thus light strikes the second lens with a vergence of (1/–0.20) –5.00D and forms an image 33cm behind the second lens (–5 + (+8) = +3.00, 100/+3.00 = +33cm). Transverse magnification for the second lens alone is –5.00D/3.00D or –1.66. The total magnification is the product of the individual magnification –1.66 x –0.25 = 0.42.

f. Axial Magnification = M_1 X M_2

Axial magnification (Figure 37) is used when talking about objects that do not occupy a single plane (3D objects). Axial magnification is the distance, along the optical axis, between the two image planes divided by the distance between the two object planes (extreme anterior and posterior points on the object with their conjugate image points). Axial magnification is proportional to the product of the transverse magnifications for the pair of conjugate planes at the front and back of the object.

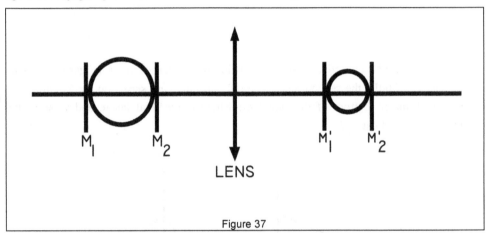

LENS

Figure 37

For objects with axial dimensions that are relatively small, M_1 and M_2 are usually very close in numerical value, which leads to the approximate formula of:

Axial Magnification = M^2

Where M is the transverse magnification for any pair of the object's conjugates.

Question: The front of a 5cm thick object is 20cm in front of a +9.00D lens. Calculate the axial magnification using both formulas.

Answer: The two faces of the object are positioned 20 and 25cm in front of the lens. From the vergence equation, the face located 20cm (U = 100/–20 = –5.00D) in front of the lens is imaged 25 cm behind the lens (U + D = V = –5 + (+9) = +4D, v = 100/+4 = +25cm). The magnification = image distance/object distance = +25/–20 = –1.25X.

The other side of the object located 25cm (100/–25 = –4.00D) from the lens is imaged at 20cm (U + D = V = –4 + (+9) = +5D, v = 100/+5 = +20cm) behind the lens with a magnification of 20/–25 = –0.8

Using the approximation formula, the axial magnification is either $(-1.25)^2 = 1.56$ or $(-0.8)^2 = 0.64$, depending on which plane we choose.

Using the exact formula, the axial magnification is –0.8 x –1.25 = 1.00

Question: An example of the importance of axial magnification is the evaluation of optic nerve cupping using indirect ophthalmoscopy. The cup can be evaluated using a +20.00D lens, but a +14.00D lens markedly improves the evaluation. What is the axial magnification of a 20D versus a 14D-condensing lens?

Answer: Lateral magnification produced through the indirect ophthalmoscope is the ratio of the total refracting power of the eye (60D) to the power of the condensing lens. The 14.00 diopter lens gives a slightly larger transverse magnification (60/20 = 3X versus 60/14 = 4.286X), but a significantly larger axial magnification because axial magnification increases as the square of transverse magnification ($3X^2 = 9X$ versus $4.286X^2 = 18.37X$). Larger axial magnification increases the distance between the optic nerve rim and the base of the cup in the aerial image, improving assessment of the cup.

g. Effective Magnification = $M_e = dF$ ← *doped needs to be at focal point of lens*

Where d = reference distance in meters to the object (image is formed at infinity)

If d = 25cm than $M_e = F/4$

If d = 40cm than $M_e = F/2.5$

Question: A +24.00D lens is used as a hand held magnifier with the patient viewing an object that is 50cm from the eye and at the focal point of the lens. How much larger do things appear to the patient?

Answer: d = 0.50m, F= +24.00D, $M_e = dF = 0.50(24) = 12X$

This indicates that closer working distances result in less effective magnification.

h. Rated Magnification = $M_r = F/4$

Assumes that the individual can accommodate up to 4.00 diopters when doing close work which gives d = 25cm (25cm is the standard reference distance used when talking about magnification).   ← *dist doiect is from person. Magnifier is moved within that 25 cm until doiect is at its focal point*

Question: A simple lens magnifier to be used as a low vision device is marked 5X (reference plane at 25cm). What would you expect to find when you measure the lens on a lensometer?

Answer: M = F/4 = 5 = F/4, F = 20D

Question: A view of the retina is obtained through an indirect ophthalmoscope, using a 30-diopter lens. The observer is 40cm from the arial image. What is the perceived lateral magnification?

Answer: 1.25x

Explanation: Lateral magnification produced through the indirect ophthalmoscope is the ratio of the total refracting power of the eye (60D) to the power of the condensing lens (30D), assuming the standard reference distance for magnification of 25cm from the observer to the arial image. If the distance is greater than 25cm, the lateral magnification is multiplied by the ratio of the standard reference distance, 25cm, to the distance in question, 40cm.

60/30D = 2x magnification at 25cm (2 x 25cm/40cm) = 1.25x magnification

i. Conventional Magnification = $M_c = dF + 1$

The underlying assumption in this equation is that the patient is "supplying" one unit (1X) of magnification

Question: Which patient needs more magnification and which patient needs the stronger lens? Patient A wants to read 1M print and has a near acuity of 2M using a +5.00 diopter add at 20cm. Patient B also wants to read 1M and has an acuity of 3M with a +2.50 diopter add at 40cm.

Answer: Patient A reads 2M print and wants to read 1M print, therefore, 2M/1M = 2x magnification. F_s needed is +5D X 2 = +10.00 diopters.

Patients B needs 3M/1M or 3x magnification and has F_s of +2.5x3 = +7.5D. Even though Patient B needs 1 ½ times the amount of magnification Patient A does, (3M versus 2M to start) he actually requires a weaker lens than Patient A does.

This apparent paradox in magnification is because we are comparing apples to oranges when we use different distances. To compensate for different viewing distances, change patient B's working distance to 20cm, the same as patient A. He would then see 1.5M print using a 5.00 diopter add for the 20cm working distance. 1.5M/1M = 1.5x times 5 diopters which = 7.5 diopters of magnification needed.

j. Magnification Ratings

Some companies use F/4 (Rated Magnification) while others use (F/4) + 1 (Conventional Magnification) to determine magnification strength for their magnifiers. This is why dioptric power, which is an absolute value and is the same under all conditions, is a better way to discuss the magnification needs of an individual.

k. Determining Needed Magnification

- Magnification needs are based on the initial reference value and the desired final value. Clinically, it is the entrance acuity divided by the goal acuity (VA/VA).

28. Telescopes   *light entering · exiting is parallel*

Telescopes are afocal optical systems consisting of two lenses, separated in space, in air. There are two types of telescopic systems, Keplerian and Galilean.

a. Keplerian telescopes (+) (+)

Keplerian telescopes have a weak (+) objective lens and a strong (+) eyepiece lens. (Figure 38)

The lenses are separated by the sum of their focal lengths. Keplerian (astronomical) telescopes form an inverted image so they require an erecting lens or prisms to make it a Terrestrial telescope.

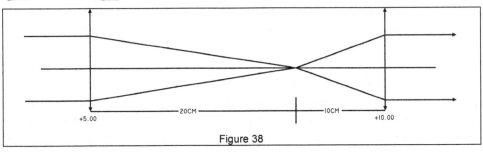

Figure 38

b. Galilean telescopes (+) (−)

Galilean telescopes (Figure 39) have a weak (+) objective lens and a strong (−) eyepiece lens. The lenses are separated by the difference of their focal lengths. Galilean telescopes form an erect/upright image.

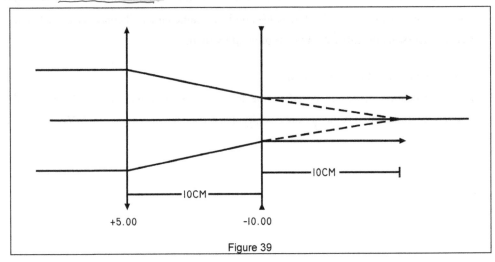

Figure 39

The *angular magnification* of a telescope is equal to the power of the eyepiece divided by the power of the objective.

$$M_{A \text{ Telescope}} = (-) F_E/F_O$$

- The eyepiece in the Galilean telescope has a negative power. Therefore, the magnification given by the equation above is positive, indicating an upright image.
- Keplerian telescopes have both positive objective and eyepiece lenses; the magnification is negative, indicating an inverted image.
- With any telescope, the secondary focal point of the first lens must coincide with the primary focal point of the second lens. With Galilean telescopes, the second lens is minus and so the primary focal point is virtual.
- Galilean telescopes have several practical advantages for low vision work. The image is upright, without the need for image erecting prisms and the device is shorter. Galilean telescopes typically are 2, 3 or 4x in strength, inexpensive, light, and have a large exit pupil, which makes centering less difficult.
- 4x telescopes and stronger are usually Keplerian in design which gives an optically superior image, but are more expensive with a smaller exit pupil requiring better centering and aiming. Keplerian binoculars, contain prisms to erect the otherwise inverted image.
- Galilean telescopes used as surgical loupes, require an add to be combined with the objective lens. The field size is far smaller than that obtained with bifocal spectacles.
- Telescopic loupes can produce asthenopia with any type of refractive error. If binocular loupes are not aligned properly, vertical or horizontal phorias can be induced. Adopting a working distance too far inside the focal distance of the "add" can require excessive accommodation, even for a myope.
- When viewing a near object through an afocal telescope, the telescope acts as a vergence multiplier. The approximate accommodation required is given by $A_{oc} = M^2U$, where A_{oc} = vergence at the eyepiece = accommodation, U = object vergence at the objective = $1/u$, M = the magnification of the telescope.

Accom needed with afocal Telescope

Aocular = $M^2 U$

20 cm

Question: How far apart must a +5D lens and a –10D lens be placed to form a Galilean (afocal) telescope?

Answer: With any telescope, the secondary focal point of the first lens must coincide with the primary focal point of the second lens. With Galilean telescopes, the second lens is minus and so the primary focal point is virtual. To make the secondary focal point (20cm) of the plus lens coincide with the virtual primary focal point of the minus lens (10cm), the lenses must be separated by 20 – 10 = 10cm.

Question: You are a –5.00D spectacle corrected myope stranded on a small island with your significant other. Unfortunately, your companion has broken your glasses (which had an 11mm vertex distance). The only lens available to you is a –55D Hruby lens, which your companion had.

a) How many cm from the eye should you hold the lens to fully correct your refractive error?

Answer: a) first, locate the far point of your eye. The far point of the lens is 0.211m in front of the eye (F = 1/–5 which equals 0.20m + 0.011m vertex distance = 0.211m = 211mm). The Hruby lens has a power of –55D which means, its focal point is 1/55 which equals 0.018m or 18mm away from the lens. To correct the refractive error, the focal point of the lens should coincide with the far point of the eye. Therefore, it should be 18mm away from the far point or 211 – 18 = 193mm in front of the eye.

20 cm

Question: Why would you not be able to read the 20/20 line with this correction?

Answer: b) The problem is magnification. This configuration turns the combination of the eye and its corrective lens into a reverse Galilean telescope, where the eyepiece is approximately +5D (the extra power of the myopic eye) and the objective lens is

–55D. The resulting magnification is (–) 5/–55, which equals 0.1x. Thus, the 20/20 line, while in focus, subtends 1/10 of the angle it would in the eye of an emmetrope. Therefore, the best distance acuity obtainable is only about 20/200, assuming an otherwise normal eye.

It should be noted that properly corrected patients with high myopia might not be able to read 20/20 through their spectacle lenses even in the absence of other pathology. This is because the longer axial length commonly found in higher amounts of myopia, results in greater separation of the photoreceptors, which decrease the visual potential of the eye.

Question: You and a stowaway are ship wrecked on a lost island with your trial lens set, but only a few lenses survive the shipwreck. Your are left with a –20D, +4D, +5D, and a +20D. You build a viewing device to search the horizon for ships using the –20D and the +4D lens. The stowaway, Dr. Smith, uses the +20D and the +5D lens. Dr. Smith complains that his viewing device is inferior.

a) What did each of you build?
b) How did you position the lenses?
c) Why is Dr. Smith plotting to steal your telescope?

Answer: You use the –20D lens as the eyepiece and the +4D lens as the objective lens of a Galilean telescope. The secondary focal point of the plus lens should coincide with the primary focal point of the minus lens, thus the lenses are 25cm – 5cm = 20cm apart. Dr. Smith built a second telescope (astronomical) using the +20.00 diopter lens as the eyepiece and the +5D lens as the objective. The secondary focal point of the objective lens needs to coincide with the primary focal point of the eye piece lens, so he positions them 5 cm + 20 cm = 25 cm apart.

Dr. Smith does not like having to stretch his arms the additional 5cm.

Question: Which telescope above will provide more magnification?

Answer: The angular magnification of a telescope is equal to the power of the eyepiece divided by the power of the objective. Magnification of the Galilean telescope is (–)–20/4 = 5x. The magnification of the astronomical telescope is (–) 20/5 = –4x. Therefore, Dr. Smith's telescope will provide less magnification.

Question: Will the telescopes have an erect or inverted image?

Answer: The Galilean telescope will produce an upright image of the, hopefully approaching ships, while Dr. Smith's astronomical telescope will produce an inverted image.

Question: How is the Galilean telescope modified when used as a surgical loupe?

Answer: The binocular surgical loupe is just a short Galilean telescope with an add to bring the working distance in from infinity. Powerful lenses are used so that the tube length of the telescope is kept to a minimum. A +25D object, combined with a –50D eyepiece, would provide 2x magnification. The additional add needed to focus the telescope at near is the reciprocal of the working distance in meters. Example: for a 25cm working distance, the add would be 100/25 = 4D.

Question:
a)   How long is the 2x Galilean telescope described above?
b)   What if it were made using a +5D objective lens and a –10D eyepiece lens?

Answer:
a) The focal length of the –50D lens is 1/50 =2cm. The +25D lens has a 100/25 = 4cm focal length. Thus, the telescope is 4 – 2 = 2cm long.
b) The +5/–10 telescope is 20 – 10 = 10cm long.

Question: You are working with a 2x afocal Galilean telescope that is fabricated with a +8D objective lens. We know that the ocular lens must be –16D and the 2 lenses are separated by 6.25cm (objective lens 1/8 = 12.5cm, ocular lens 1/16 = 6.25cm, tube length = 12.5 – 6.25 = 6.25cm).

When viewing at infinity by an uncorrected 4D hyperope, the ocular has an effective power of?

Answer: +4 is needed to correct for the hyperopic refractive error. This power must be taken from the ocular lens of the telescope and so the effective power of the ocular lens becomes –16 – 4 = – 20D. (The –20D effective ocular lens combined with the +4D correction lens gives us the –16D the ocular lens of the telescope actually has).

Question: For the telescope to remain afocal, the tube length must be?

Answer: The objective lens focal length is still 12.5cm, ocular lens is now 1/20 = 5cm. Therefore 12.5 – 5 = 7.5cm

Question: What is the telescopic power now?

Answer: $M_{A\ Telescope} = (-)F_E/F_O = (-)-20/8 = 2.5x$

Question: When viewed by an uncorrected 4D myope, the ocular has an effective power of?

Answer: The uncorrected –4D of the eye must act as a correcting lens so the ocular now has an effected power of –16 + 4 = –12D. (The –12D effective ocular lens combined with the –4D correction lens gives us the –16D the ocular lens of the telescope actually has).

Question: To make the telescope afocal, the tube length must be?

Answer: The objective lens focal length is still 12.5cm, ocular lens is now 1/12 = 8.33cm. Therefore 12.5 – 8.33 = 4.17cm.

Question: What is the telescopic power now?

Answer: $M_{A \, Telescope} = -F_E/F_O = (-)-12/8 = 1.5x.$

Question: An afocal Keplerian telescope has an objective lens that is +7D and an eyepiece lens that is +17.50D. What is the separation between the lenses?

Answer: The focal length of the objective lens is 1/7 = 14.3cm. The focal length of the eyepiece lens is 1/17.5 = 5.7cm. Therefore, the lens separation is 14.3 + 5.7 = 20cm

Question: What is the power of the telescope now?

Answer: $M_{A \, Telescope} = (-)F_E/F_O = (-)17.5/7 = -2.5x$

Question: A patient uses a focusable 2x Keplerian telescope that has a +8D objective lens. What is the power and tube length of the afocal telescope when used by an emmetropic patient and focused for distance viewing?

Answer: The power is 2x because it is being used by an emmetrope.

The eyepiece lens power would be +16D

$(M_{A \, Telescope} = (-)F_E/F_O = (-)X/8 = -2x)$

To find the tube length, the focal length of would be 1/8 = 12.5mm for the objective lens and 1/16 = 6.25mm for the eyepiece lens. Therefore, the tube length would be 12.5 + 6.25 = 18.75mm.

Question: When used by a 4D hyperope in a similar fashion?

Answer: For the uncorrected 4D hyperope, the eyepiece lens now has an effective power of 16 – 4 = 12D. (The +12D effective ocular lens combined with the +4D correction lens gives us the +16D the ocular lens of the telescope actually has). The power of the telescope would become (–) 12/8 = –1.5x. The tube length would be 20.83mm. (1/12 = 8.33mm + 12.5 = 20.83mm)

Question: When used by a 4D myope in a similar fashion?

Answer: For the uncorrected 4D myope, the eyepiece lens now has an effective power of 16 + 4 = 20D. (The +20D effective ocular lens combined with the –4D correction lens gives us the +16D the ocular lens of the telescope actually has). The power of the telescope would be (–)20/8 = –2.5x. The tube length would be 17.5mm (1/20 = 5mm + 12.5mm = 17.5)

Question: A focusable Galilean telescope with a +20D objective lens with a –40D ocular lens is dispensed to a patient for a variety of tasks.

a) What is the magnification of the telescope at distance?

Answer: M = (–)–40/20 = 2x

b) What tube length is required for viewing distance objects?

Answer: 1/20 = 5cm, 1/40 = 2.5cm, 5 – 2.5 = 2.5cm

c) What is the tube length required for viewing numbers that are 50cm away in an elevator?

Answer: The objective power would now be +20 + (–2) = +18D. 100/+18 = +5.55, +5.55 – 2.5 = 3.05cm.

Important to remember – 20 inches = 50 cm. To find the vergences when working in inches, use the formula V = 40/distance (inches) = 100/distance (cm)

Question: A 3x afocal Galilean telescope has a separation between the objective and ocular lens of 2cm. When viewing an object 25cm in front of the objective lens, what power reading cap would eliminate the need to accommodate for this target distance?

Answer: 100/25 = +4D

Question: A patient with vision loss needs a 10D add to read the text on a computer monitor but the 10cm working distance is too close. He wants to work at a 25cm distance. What theoretical telescope and reading cap combination would be needed?

Answer: 25/10 = 2.5x, 100/25 = +4D, therefore you would need a 2.5x telescope with a +4D reading cap.

Question: What is the equivalent lens that should be prescribed to replace a 4x telescope with a +2.50D reading cap (F_{RC}) so the patient has the same resolution ability through the lens that he has through the telemicroscopic system?

Answer: F_e = (F_{RC}) (power of telescope) = 2.5D (4) = 10D

Question: If a patient is able to read enlarged sheet music with a 3x telescope and a cap focus for 16 inches, what telescope and cap are needed to read the same sheet music set at 32 inches?

Answer: 32/16 = 2x additional magnification, 40/32 = 1.25D, Therefore you would need a 6x telescope with 1.25D cap

29. Aniseikonia

Aniseikonia…. "may be due to differences in the size of the optical images on the retina or may be anatomically determined by a different distribution in spacing of the retinal elements". (Duke-Elder, 1963)

Aniseikonia is a term coined by Dr. Walter Lancaster in 1932. It means literally "not equal images (either size, shape, or both)" from the two eyes, as perceived by the patient and is one of the problems most frequently associated with the correction of anisometropia with spectacles. It is an anomaly of the binocular visual process that affects the patient's perceptual judgment. The most common cause is the differential magnification inherent in the spectacle correction of Anisometropia. This difference in magnification produces different sized retinal images. Approximately 1/3 of the cases of aniseikonia are predicted from anisometropia. Aniseikonia is more commonly caused by unequal refractive errors common in conditions such as monocular aphakia or pseudophakic surprises. However, it is also found with retinal problems and occipital lobe lesions. Aniseikonia occurs in 5-10% of the population with only 1-3% having symptoms.

The perception of an image size disparity between the two eyes is due to the image on the retina not falling on corresponding retinal points. The ocular image is the final impression received in the higher cortical centers, involving the retinal image with modifications imposed by anatomical, physiologic, and perhaps psychological properties of the entire binocular visual apparatus. This is why there are cases of aniseikonia in individuals with emmetropia and isometropia (equal refractive errors).

In general aniseikonia is associated with a false stereoscopic localization and an apparent distortion of objects in space. Aniseikonia can be the cause of asthenopia, diplopia, suppression, poor fusion, headaches, vertigo, photophobia, amblyopia, and strabismus. The differences in size may be overall, that is, the same in all meridians, or meridional, in which the difference is greatest in one meridian and least in the meridian 90° away.

Clinically, aniseikonia usually occurs when the difference in image size between the two eyes approaches 0.75%. Individuals with greater than 4-5% image size difference, have such a large disparity in image size, that they generally do not have binocularity. It is usually assumed that patients can comfortably tolerate up to 1% of aniseikonia in non-astigmatic cases.

A change in refractive correction is always accompanied by some change in the retinal image size and in the conditions under which the patient sees. The magnitude of these changes and the patient's tolerance determines whether these changes will produce symptoms of discomfort or inefficiency. Persons with normal binocular vision can readily discriminate differences in image size as low as 0.25 to 0.5 percent. For persons with normal binocular vision, a deviation of 4-5x the threshold of discrimination is usually considered significant.

Aniseikonia can be noted when a patient, for the sake of comfort, prefers to use one eye for reading or watching moving objects. If an individual can learn to rely on non-stereoscopic, rather than stereoscopic clues, they may be able to avoid irritation from aniseikonia, even when it is present.

Aniseikonic patients may see an apparent slant of level surfaces, such as tabletops and floors. The effect is more pronounced with objects on the surfaces, for instance, with an irregular pattern carpet on the floor. For high levels of cylinder correction, spherical equivalents may help reduce the aniseikonia.

- The magnification for flat trial lens case cylinders is approximately 1.5% per diopter.

- The uncorrected refractive myopic eye will have a larger image by 1.5% per diopter and the uncorrected refractive hyperopic eye will have a smaller image by 1.5% per diopter. This holds for anisometropia primarily of refractive origin.

- The corrected refractive myopic eye will have a smaller image by 1.5% per diopter and the corrected refractive hyperopic eye will have a larger image by 1.5% per diopter. This holds for anisometropia primarily of refractive origin.

- However, since anisometropia may be partially axial, an estimate of 1% per diopter is more clinically useful.

When considering axial versus refractive anisometropia:
- If the amount of anisometropia is > 2D – assume it to be axial.
- If the amount of anisometropia is < 2D or is in cylinder only – assume it to be refractive.

Spectacle correction of astigmatism produces meridional aniseikonia with accompanying distortion of the binocular spatial sense. Anisometropia is commonly stated to be present if the difference in the refractive correction is 2.00D or more either spherical or astigmatic. However, smaller differences than 2.00D may be significant.

When prescribing aniseikonic lenses, it is important to realize that the size and shape of the final image does not matter, it is only important that the images of each eye match each other. For this reason, instead of magnifying the image of one eye, it may be easier to minify the image of another. This may allow for a more cosmetically acceptable spectacles, or at least lenses that are easier to manufacture, and therefore, less costly.

a. Cylindrical Corrections

Cylindrical corrections in spectacle lenses produce distortion. This is a problem of aniseikonia, which may be solved by prescribing iseikonic spectacle corrections. *Iseikonia* is when perceived images are the same size. Iseikonic spectacle corrections may be complicated and expensive and the vast majority of practitioners prefer to prescribe cylinders according to cylinder judgment using guidelines that have evolved over the years. Remember the reason for intolerance of an astigmatic spectacle correction is distortion caused by meridional magnification which is more poorly tolerated. Unequal magnification of the retinal image in the various meridians produced monocular distortion manifested by tilted lines or altered shapes of objects. The monocular distortion by itself is rarely a problem. The effect is too small.

Oblique meridional aniseikonia causes a rotary deviation between fused images of vertical lines in the two eyes. The maximum tilting of vertical lines is called the *Declination Error*. The maximum declination error occurs when the corrected cylinder axis is at 45 or 135°, but even under these conditions, each diopter of correcting cylinder power produces only about 0.4° of tilt. This problem occurs more often with plus cylinder lenses which is why most spectacle lenses are now made in the minus cylinder form. Clinically significant problem begin to occur when the declination approaches 0.3%. Minor degrees of monocular distortion can produce major alterations in binocular spatial perception.

The *Total Magnification of a Lens (M_T)* is found by adding the magnification from its power (M_P) and the magnification from its shape (M_S). Therefore, total magnification $M_T = M_P + M_S$.

Magnification from Power (M$_P$) is dependent on the dioptric power of the lens (D$_V$) and its vertex distance (H). If H is measured in cm, the relationship is M$_P$ = D$_V$H. From this formula, we see that moving a lens away from the eye increases the magnification of a plus lens and the minification of a minus lens. Moving a lens toward the eye (decreasing the vertex distance) decreases the magnification of a plus lens and the minification of a minus lens. These effects are especially notable with higher powered lenses.

Examples

+10.00D lens @ 10mm and 15mm vertex distance

@ 10mm, M$_P$ = D$_V$H = +10.00 x 1.0 = +10

@ 15mm, M$_P$ = D$_V$H = +10.00 x 1.5 = +15

−10.00D lens @ 10 and 15 mm vertex distance

@ 10mm, M$_P$ = D$_V$H = −10.00 x 1.0 = −10

@ 15mm, M$_P$ = D$_V$H = −10.00 x 1.5 = −15

For spectacle lenses remember, as you move a lens closer to the eye, you must add plus power to the lens. Therefore remember *CAP = Closer Add Plus.*

Magnification from Shape (M$_S$) is dependent on the curvature of the front surface of the lens D$_1$ and the center thickness of the lens t. The 1.5 in the following equation is the index of refraction (approximately) of glass or plastic. M$_S$ = D$_1$ (t$_{cm}$/1.5). Therefore, the more curved the lens, the larger the D$_1$ and the more magnification from shape the lens have. Also, the thicker the lens (t), the more magnification from shape.

Examples

Front curve of a +2.00D lens is +2.00D and +6.00D, Thickness is 2mm.

M$_S$ = D$_1$ (t$_{cm}$/1.5) = +2.00(0.2/1.5) = +0.27

M$_S$ = D$_1$ (t$_{cm}$/1.5). = +6.00(0.2/1.5) = +0.80

Front curve of a +2.00D lens is +2.00D and +6.00D, Thickness is 4mm.

M$_S$ = D$_1$ (t$_{cm}$/1.5) = +2.00(0.4/1.5) = +0.53

M$_S$ = D$_1$ (t$_{cm}$/1.5). = +6.00(0.4/1.5) = +1.60

Magnification may be reduced by making the front surface power of a lens less positive.

Decreasing center thickness also decreases magnification.

However, a change in either the front curve or the thickness of the lens will also cause the vertex distance (h) to be changed so that the magnification from the power factor (M$_P$) is also affected. If the front curve is changed to give the magnification or minification needed, the back curve must also be changed to maintain the same power of the lens.

If, for example, the front curve is increased, the back curve must also be increased, which increases the vertex distance. If the front curve is flattened, the back curve must be flattened, which causes the vertex distance to decrease. If center thickness is increased to increase the magnification of the lens, but the front curve is left the same, the increase moves the back surface closer to the eye by the amount of the increase, therefore decreasing the vertex distance. On the other hand, it the center thickness is decreased, but the front curve is left the same, the decrease causes the vertex distance to be increased by that amount.

For further review on this subject, go to the *THILL Aniseikonia Worksheet* in Duane's Clinical Ophthalmology (Lippincott Williams & Wilkins).

Contact lenses may provide a better solution than spectacles in most patients with anisometropia, particularly children, where fusion may be possible, because it gives the least change in image size from the uncorrected state in refractive ametropia.

30. Multifocal Design

Bifocals are made in two different ways. (Figure 40) One piece and fused lenses.

The one-piece type is made from one piece of glass or plastic. The lens surface is ground with two different curvatures. The shorter radius of curvature in the bifocal area creates the additional power. Fusing two different types of glass together makes fused bifocals. Each type of glass has a different index of refraction, which is not possible with plastic lenses. The segment button has a higher refractive index (flint n = 1.7) than the basic lens (crown n = 1.523).

Most flat top fused segments are designed with the optical center 4 mm below the segment top and produce only a very small amount of image jump (see below). Larger, flat top segments are similar to an executive bifocal, in that they will have little to no image jump.

ROUND TOP

USUAL SEGMENT DIAMETER 22CM
(FROM 13.22MM)

FLAT TOP

SEGMENT DIAMETER
20 22 25 28 35 45 MM

CURVED TOP

RIBBON SEGMENTS

THIS FUSED BIFOCAL IS
DESIGNED TO PERMIT
DISTANCE VISION VIEWING
BELOW THIS SEGMENT

ONE-PIECE BIFOCALS

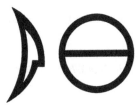

SPLIT LENS (OR "BENJAMIN FRANKLIN")
BIFOCAL CORRECTION FOR ASTIGMATISM
IS GROUND ON THE CONCAVE SURFACE.

ULTEX TYPE BIFOCALS IN SEGMENT DIAMETERS

ULTEX B   22MM
ULTEX E   32MM
ULTEX A   38MM
ULTEX AL 38MM (UP TO 33MM HIGH)
ASTIGMATISM CORRECTION IS GROUND ON
THE CONVEX SURFACES

FUSED BIFOCALS

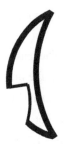

BARIUM
CROWN GLASS
(N=1.523)

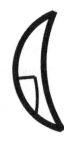

FLINT GLASS BUTTON
(N=1.654)

Figure 40

a. *Image Jump* is produced by the sudden introduction of the prismatic power at the top of a bifocal segment. The object the individual sees in the inferior field suddenly jumps upward when the eye turns down to look at it. If the optical center of the segment is at the top of the segment, there is no image jump. Image jump is worse in glasses with a round top bifocal, because the optical center of the bifocal is farther from the distance lens optical center. A flat top bifocal is better because the optical center of the bifocal is close to the distance optical center.

b. *Image Displacement* is the prismatic effect induced by the combination of the bifocal type and the power of the distance lens prescription in the reading position. Image displacement is more bothersome than image jump for most people. Most bifocal corrected presbyopes read through a point about 10 mm below the optical center of their distance lenses. If that position is also at the bifocal segment's optical center, as in most fused flat top bifocals, the bifocal segment produces no prismatic effect at all. The prismatic effect that is there is induced by the distance lens correction, not the segment. However, if the optical center of the bifocal segment is located below or above the reading position, the bifocal will contribute to image displacement at the reading position. The total prismatic displacement will be the sum of that produced by the bifocal and that induced by the distance lens.

A flat top lens is essentially a base up prism, whereas a round top lens is a base down prism at the normal reading spot, 10 mm below the optical center of the lens. A myopic distance lens has base down prismatic power in the reading position; thus, *image displacement* is worsened with a round top lenses. The prism effects are additive. Similarly, a hyperopic spectacle lens is a base up prism in the reading position; thus a flat top lens makes image displacement an issue.

Most individuals will physiologically adapt, or learn to fuse small vertical deviations. If they cannot, there are several ways to compensate for the problem including, using contact lenses instead of spectacles, prescribing dissimilar segments, or providing "slab-off" prism.

In the past, slab-off prism (base up) was added to the spectacle lens that had the most minus or least plus correction for distance. Now, with modern plastic lenses, slab-off prism is taken off the mold, effectively adding base down prism to the most plus or less minus lens. This is called "reverse slab". Slab off is fabricated by way of bicentric grinding which creates two optical centers in the lens. One optical center is for the distance correction and the other is for the reading correction of the lens.

Question: If a patient comes in wearing glasses: OD +2.00, OS –2.00, and complains of vertical diplopia when reading. Both eyes are reading 5 mm down from the optical center. How much slab-off do you prescribe?

Answer: 2.00 prism diopters base up OS. A slab-off prism is always put in front of the more minus eye because slab off provides base up prism. In this example, the right eye will have induced 1.00 prism diopter base up and the left eye will have induced 1.00 prism diopter base down.

Question: Should a hyperope use a round top or a flat top bifocal?

Answer: A plus lens will have significant image displacement with a flat top lens. Image displacement is lessened with a round top lens. Although image jump will be present, it is less disturbing than image displacement.

Question: Should a myope use a flat top or a round top bifocal?

Answer: A round top lens has significant image displacement with a minus lens. A flat top lens minimizes image displacement and image jump for a myope.

Question: What is the induced prism for an individual wearing +5.00D OU, when reading at the usual reading position of 2mm in and 8mm down from the optical center of his lenses?

Answer: PD = hF, therefore,

vertically +5.00D x 0.8 = 4PD BU per eye

horizontally +5.00D x 0.2 = 1PD BO per eye

Question: What vertically compensating prism is needed for an individual wearing +5.00D OD and +2.00D OS when they are viewed in the normal reading position of 8mm down from the optical center of the lens?

Answer: +5.00D x 0.8 = 4PD BU and +2.00 x 0.8 = 1.6PD BU, 4–1.6 = 2.4PD BU needed for the left eye.

31. Visual Acuity Assessment

- Measures spatial resulting capacity (ability to see fine detail) of the visual system
- Allows for quantification of degree of high contrast vision loss
- Monitors stability or progression of disease and visual abilities as rehabilitation progresses
- Allows assessment of eccentric viewing postures and skills, patient motivation and scanning ability (for field loss)
- Allows teaching of basic concepts and skills (i.e., eccentric viewing)
- Is the basis for determining initial magnification requirements
- Verify eligibility for tasks such as driving
- Verify eligibility as "legally blind"
- Inaccurate acuity testing underestimates ability

Factors to consider when measuring VA include; contrast of chart, lighting, number of optotypes at each acuity level, spacing of targets, difficulty of targets used (letters, numbers, pictures), single targets versus words (or multiple digits) versus continuous text, eccentric viewing postures, expressive as well as receptive language skills and cognitive level. The best quantification of visual acuity is obtained when using appropriate charts.

It is important to accurately measure visual acuity to determine if your refraction/plan of care is helping. For this reason, do not use "counts fingers" if at all possible. If the patient can see fingers, they can read the larger figures on the chart, if the chart is brought closer.

If you must use "counts fingers", note the distance at which the patient can count your fingers. Most fingers are equivalent in size to a 200 (60) size letter. Therefore, CF at 3 feet (1 meter) is equivalent to 3/200 (1/60) = 20/1300 (6/360).

If the patient's visual acuity is reduced to the point where they can only see "hand motions", note which quadrant(s) and at what distance? If the patient can only see light, do they have "light perception with projection" versus just "light perception"? If yes, in which quadrant(s) and at what distance?

Shorter test distances allow for greater accuracy when measuring lower levels of acuity

Typical starting test distances are 5 of 10 feet or 2 to 4 meters, depending on the chart used. Remember to account for accommodative demands at closer distances.

81

Record the visual acuity as actual test distance over size of character read.

For a Snellen or Feinbloom chart, the test distance in feet becomes the numerator, and the size of the number read (noted in foot size) is the denominator

Example: 400 size optotype @ 10 feet = 10/400, 80 size optotype @ 5 feet = 5/80

For the ETDRS chart, measure at 1, 2 or 4 meters

Use the testing distance as the numerator, and the M size of the letters read as the denominator. M size is given in the far left column. The next column gives the conversion to Snellen equivalent (not the letter size). For example, when testing at 2 meters and the patient reads the 32M line (160 Snellen equivalent), the acuity is recorded as 2/32 = 20/320.

During measurement of visual acuity, the clinician should evaluate eccentric viewing techniques demonstrated by the patient.

Near Acuity Measurement & Charts
- The M unit chart was developed by Bailey in 1978. The International Council of Ophthalmology as well as the International Society for Low Vision Research and Rehabilitation recommends metric acuity testing, because it is the most accurate and reproducible test available.
- Testing distance must be measured and recorded
- The designation of letters signs (e.g., 1M, 2M) indicates the distance in which the print is equivalent in angular size to a 20/20 optotype. Example: 1M print subtends 5 minutes of arc at 1 meter

Near Acuity Charts

ETDRS near charts
- Like distance version, has a logarithmic progression in sizes, with proportional spacing of letters and rows which allows the task to remain constant at different distances

Lighthouse "Game" & "Number" cards
- Words and triple digit numbers
- Allows assessment of "crowding" as well as cognitive influences in reading difficulties

Sloan continuous text reading cards

- Continuous text cards of appropriate reading level will provide a more accurate measure of reading ability than single optotype acuities

Jaeger Acuity

- Least desirable letter-size designation (Source: International Council of Ophthalmology and the American Academy of Ophthalmology)
- Jaeger numbers are a printer's designation that refer to the boxes in the print shop in Vienna where Jaeger selected his print samples in 1854
- The print boxes are not proportional to the letter size
- System has never been standardized
- Print size is not the same from one test card or chart to another

Recording near acuity

Near visual acuity is recorded as testing distance in meters over M-size letter read. Can also be recorded as M-sized read at what testing distance. For example, if a 4M letter is read at 40 cm, the acuity is recorded as 0.40/4M or 4M @ 40cm.

Use of the M system also facilitates calculation of addition power (i.e., the dioptric power required to focus at a specific metric distance). For example, if a patient reads 0.40/4M and wants to read 1M print, they must hold the material 4x closer. Therefore, .40/4M = X/1M. X = .10M or 10cm. The lens that focuses at this distance is 100/10 = +10D

Types of Visual Acuity Testing

a. Minimum Visible Acuity: measures brightness discrimination; the person's ability to detect small differences in the brightness of two light sources. Minimum visible acuity is determined by the brightness of the object relative to its background illumination as opposed to the visual angle subtend by the object.

b. Minimum Perceptible Acuity: measures **detection** discrimination. Minimum perceptible acuity is concerned with simple detection of objects, not their identification or naming. An example of this type of acuity testing is determining if a child can see and grasp a small candy bead held in the examiner's hand.

c. Minimum Separable Acuity: measures the **resolution** threshold, or smallest visual angle at which two separate objects can be discriminated. Landolt C, and grating acuity are examples of minimum separable tasks.

d. Vernier Acuity (hyper acuity): a precise form of visual discrimination still under study. Hyper acuity has been coined to classify the high precision (within a few seconds of arc) with which vernier alignment task can be performed. This level of precision is well above resolution or recognition acuity thresholds.

e. Minimum Legible Acuity: measures the individual's ability to **recognize** progressively smaller objects (letters, numbers or objects) called optotypes. The angle that the smallest recognized letter or symbol subtends on the retina is a measure of visual acuity. This type of acuity testing is used most often clinically.

f. Snellen Acuity uses a notation in which the numerator is the testing distance (in feet or meters) and the denominator is the distance at which a letter subtends the standard visual angle of 5 minutes. A 20/20 letter (6/6 in meters) subtends an angle of 5 minutes when viewed at 20 feet (6 meters). Each leg and space of the "E" is 1 minute (1/60 degrees) = 0.017 degrees of visual angle. The 20/20 "E" viewed on a chart meant to be viewed at 20 feet is about 9 mm tall. Each leg and space between the legs is about 1.7 mm tall. For the Landolt "C", the opening in the "C" is about 1.75 mm (1 minute of arc).

Question: How many minutes does the "E" on the 20/20 line of the Snellen eye chart subtend?

Answer: 5 minutes at 20 feet. Snellen eye chart measures the minimum legible acuity.

Question: What is the optimum size of pinhole used to measure "pinhole acuity"?

Answer: The optimum size is 1.2 mm. Larger pinholes do not effectively neutralize refractive error and smaller pinholes markedly increase diffraction and decrease the amount of light entering the eye.

32. Contrast Sensitivity

Contrast indicates the variation in brightness of an object. When an eye chart uses perfectly black ink on perfectly white paper, 100% contrast is achieved. Acuity charts approximate 100% contrast. Acuity charts are helpful for characterizing central visual acuity. However, they are less helpful for examining visual function away from fixation.

Contrast sensitivity is tested using alternating light and dark bars at varying intensity. The number of light bands per-unit length or per-unit angle is called the spatial frequency. During clinical testing of contrast sensitivity, patients are presented with targets of various spatial frequencies and peak contrasts. The minimum resolvable contrast is the contrast threshold. The reciprocal of the contrast threshold is defined as the contrast sensitivity, and the manner in which contrast sensitivity changes as a function of the spatial frequencies of the target is called the contrast sensitivity function.

Contrast sensitivity can be tested with sine wave gratings presented using either charts or video gratings. Because standard Snellen acuity charts test only the higher spatial frequency (30 cycles per degree), they do not provide an accurate picture of an individual's visual functioning, particularly when the individual has an ocular disease.

Acuity charts provide us with a quantitative assessment of visual functioning while contrast sensitivity charts provide us with a qualitative assessment of visual functioning. Contrast sensitivity testing is similar to current audiological testing which assesses an individual's ability to hear various tones and frequencies.

Contrast sensitivity testing can detect changes in visual function at times when Snellen visual acuity is normal. This can occur when corneal pathology, cataracts, glaucoma and various other ocular diseases are present.

33. Jackson Cross Cylinder (JCC)

Cross cylinders are combinations of two cylinders whose powers are numerically equal and of opposite sign and whose axes are perpendicular to each other. The Jackson Cross Cylinder is usually mounted in a ring with a handle at 45 degrees from the axis so that a twirl of the handle changes the cross cylinder to a second position.

Example: +0.25x90/–0.25x180 to –0.25x90/+0.25x180

When the JCC is placed in contact with a spherocylinder, it displaces both focal lines simultaneously in opposite directions, expanding the initial Interval of Sturm in the first position and contracting it in the second. However, there will be no displacement of the Circle of Least Confusion, only the diameter of the circle will increase in the first and decrease in the second position of the JCC.

When a +/–0.50 JCC is placed on a lensometer, with the red axis at 0 and 180 degrees, the lensometer will read the power as –0.50 +1.00 x 090. But, remembering that the JCC has no spherical power, only cylindrical power. For this reason, we can more accurately write the power of the JCC as –0.50 x 180 combined with +0.50 x 90

Question: When the Jackson cross cylinder is used to define the astigmatic axis, is the handle of the lens parallel to the axis or 45 degrees from it?

Answer: Parallel. To define the astigmatic power, the handle is rotated 45 degrees to the axis. Normally, you should define the axis before the power.

34. Duochrome Test

Chromatic aberration of the eye results in green light being focused in front of the retina, yellow light at the retinal plane, and red light behind the retina. Therefore, when red is brighter, it indicates that more minus is needed to move the focus of red light further behind the retina? When green is brighter, more plus is needed to move the green light to focus further into the posterior chamber.

35. Night Myopia

Light rays at the edge of the human lens are refracted more than those at the center of the lens. Because our pupils are larger at night, more spherical aberration is present under lower light conditions. A refractive shift towards more myopia is needed to compensate for this increase in spherical aberration. Additionally, accommodation does not go to a neutral state under low light conditions. The visual system actually accommodates approximately 0.75D under low light conditions. These changes result in a need for more minus or less plus correction for those individuals, such as over the road truck drivers, who need to function with their highest visual clarity at night.

36. Ring Scotoma

Produced by the aphakic or high plus spectacle lens resulting from the prism effect induced by the peripheral edge of the lens which possesses the maximum prismatic power and creates the greatest deviation of rays.

37. Lensmaker equation

The surface power of a lens $= D_s = (n'- n)/r$, where r is in meters, n = the index of the object space (air or fluid the lens is in) and n' = the index of the lens. This is also called the refractive power or simply the power of a spherical refracting surface.

The power of a thin lens (IOL) immersed in fluid

$D_{air}/D_{fluid} = (n_{IOL} - n_{air})/(n_{IOL} - n_{fluid})$

38. IOL Power (SRK Formula)

$D_{IOL} = A - 2.5L - 0.9K$. Where D_{IOL} = recommended power for emmetropia, A = a constant (provided by manufacturers for their lenses), L = axial length in mm, K = average keratometry reading in diopters for desired ametropia. Change IOL power by 1.25 to 1.5D for each diopter of desired ametropia. Alternate formulas are needed for shorter or longer eyes.

39. Instruments

a. Lens Clock = Lens Gauge = Geneva Lens Measure

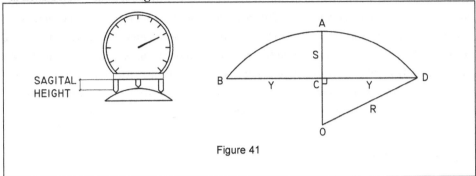

Figure 41

The lens measure, lens clock, or lens gauge has two fixed pins on the outside and in the center, a spring-loaded, movable pin. This device physically measures the sagital depth of a refracting surface and calculates the refracting power of the surface. A pointer that is activated by a system of gears indicates the position of the movable pin in relation to the fixed pins. If the instrument is placed on a flat surface, the protrusion of the central pin is equal to that of the fixed pins, with the result that the scale reading is zero. If placed on a convex surface, the protrusion of the central pin is less than that of the fixed pins, but if placed on a concave surface, the protrusion of the central pin is greater. Because the chord length (the distance between the two outer pins) has a constant value for the instrument, the position of the central pin, indicates the sagitta of the surface, which provides a direct reading of diopters of refracting power of a surface of the lens.

- The lens clock physically measures the sagital height/depth.
- The reading is in power (diopters)
- The lens clock assumes that n is in air and n' = 1.53 (crown glass)

To calculate for the lens radius (assumes that s is very small) $r = y^2/2s$ (see diagram)

To calculate true power of a single refracting surface (SRS)

$F_{true} = F_{lens\ clock} (n'_{true} - n)/(n'_{lens\ clock} - n)$

Question: What is a Geneva lens clock?

Answer: A device used to determine the base curve of the back surface of a spectacle lens. It is often used clinically to detect plus cylinder spectacle lenses in an individual who is use to minus cylinder lenses. It is specifically calibrated for the refractive index of crown glass (n = 1.53). Special lens clocks are available for plastic lenses.

Question: A lens clock measures the power of a high index plastic lens (n=−1.66) to be −5.00 diopters. Has the lens clock overestimated, underestimated or accurately determined the power of the lens?

Answer: The lens clock has underestimated the power of the surface.

$n' > 1.53$ — *clock under estimates*

$n' < 1.53$ — *over estimates clock*

Question: A lens clock is used to measure the power of a SRS where n = 1.00 and n' = 1.60.

1.   What is the true power of the SRS if the lens clock reads −10.00D?

$F_{true} = F_{lens\ clock}\ (n'_{true} - n)/(n'_{lens\ clock} - n) = -10.00D\ (1.6-1)/(1.53-1) =$
$-10.00\ (.6/.53) = -10.00D\ (1.132) = -11.32D$

2.   How much error was induced by the lens clock? $-11.32 - (-10.00) = -1.32D$

Question: A lens clock is used to measure the power of a SRS where n = 1.00 and n' = 1.498.

1.   What is the true power of the SRS if the lens clock reads −10.00D?
$F_{true} = F_{lens\ clock}\ (n'_{true} - n)/(n'_{lens\ clock} - n) = -10.00D\ (1.498-1)/(1.53-1) =$
$-10.00\ (.498/.53) = -10.00D\ (0.939) = -9.39D$

2.   How much error was induced by the lens clock? $-9.39 - (-10.00) = +0.61D$

From these examples, you see that for lenses made with indexes of refraction greater than crown glass, the lens clock will underestimate the true lens power and for those lenses with indexes of refraction less than crown glass, the lens clock will overestimate the true lens power.

b. Manual lensometer

The lensometer measures the vertex power of the lens. The vertex power is the reciprocal of the distance between the back surface of the lens and its secondary focal point. This is also known as the back focal length. For this reason, a lensometer does not really measure the focal length of a lens. The true focal lengths are measured from the principal planes, not from the lens surface. The lensometer works on the Badel principle with the addition of an astronomical telescope for precise detection of parallel rays at neutralization. The Badel principle is Knapp's law applied to lensometers.

A lensometer is really an optical bench consisting of an illuminated moveable target, a powerful fixed lens, and a telescopic eyepiece focused at infinity. The key element is the field lens that is fixed in place so that its focal point is on the back surface of the lens being analyzed. A lensometer measures the back vertex power of the spectacle lens. However, when measuring a bifocal addition, the spectacles must be turned around in the lensometer so that the front vertex power is measured. This is because the distance portion of the spectacle lenses is designed to deal with essentially parallel light. However, the bifocal addition is designed to work on diverging light, originating from a standard working distance of 40 centimeters. This diverging light from the near object is made parallel by the bifocal lens. The parallel light then enters the distance lens where it is refracted with the expected optical affect to give the patient clear vision. In this way, the bifocal exerts its effect on the light from the object before it passes through the rest of the lens. For strong bifocal corrections, there would be a significant difference in the bifocal strength measurement when using the front versus back vertex measurement. Higher bifocal powers will measure more powerful than they actually are when using the back vertex measurement instead of the front vertex measurement.

Performing Manual Lensometry

<u>**Focusing the Eyepiece**</u>

The focus of the lensometer eyepiece must be verified each time the instrument is used, to avoid erroneous readings.

1. With no lens or a Plano lens in place on the lensometer, look through the eyepiece of the instrument. Turn the power drum until the **mires** (the perpendicular cross lines), viewed through the eyepiece, are grossly out of focus.

2.   Turn the eyepiece in the plus direction to fog (blur) the target seen through the eyepiece.

3.   Slowly turn the eyepiece in the opposite direction until the target is clear, then stop turning. This procedure focuses the eyepiece.

4.   Turn the power drum to focus the mires. The mire should focus clearly at a power-drum reading of zero, which is Plano. If the mires do not focus at Plano, repeat the procedure from step 1.

Positioning the Eye Glasses

1.   Place the eye glasses on the movable spectacle table with the earpieces facing away from you. You are now prepared to read the back surface power of the lens, normally the appropriate surface from which to measure the power.

2.   While looking through the lensometer eyepiece, align the eyeglass lens so that the mires cross in the center of the target. By convention, the right lens power is measured first, followed by the left lens power.

Measuring Sphere and Cylinder Power

Plus-Cylinder Technique

1.   Turn the power drum to bring the closely spaced mires, often called the **single lines,** into sharp focus by rotating the power drum. At the same time, rotate the cylinder axis wheel to straighten the single lines where they cross the more widely spaced perpendicular oriented set of mires, often called **triple lines**.

2.   For plus cylinder measurements, the single line should focus with the least plus or most minus power.

3.   If the single lines and triple lines coming into focus at the same time, the lens is a sphere. If only the single lines focus, you have identified the sphere portion of the sphero-cylinder lens. In either case, record the power drum reading at this point as the power of the sphere.

4.   If cylinder power is present, after noting the power-drum reading for the sphere, measure cylinder power by moving the power-drum in a less minus or more plus direction to bring the triple lines into sharp focus.

5. Calculate the **difference** between the first power-drum reading for the focus single lines and the second power-drum reading for the focused triple lines, and record this figure as the plus-cylinder power of the lens.

6. Read the axis of the cylinder off the cylinder axis wheel.

Minus-Cylinder Technique

1. Turn the power drum to bring the closely spaced mires, often called the **single lines**, into sharp focus by rotating the power drum. At the same time, rotate the cylinder axis wheel to straighten the single lines where they cross the more widely spaced perpendicular oriented set of mires, often called **triple lines**.

2. For minus cylinder measurements, the single lines should focus with the most plus or least of minus power.

3. If the single lines and triple lines coming into focus at the same time, the lens is a sphere. If only the single lines focus, you have identified the sphere portion of the sphero-cylinder lens. In either case, record the power drum reading at this point as the power of the sphere.

4. If cylinder power is present, after noting the power-drum reading for the sphere, measure cylinder power by moving the power-drum in a more minus or less plus direction to bring the triple lines into sharp focus.

5. Calculate the **difference** between the first power-drum reading for the focus single lines and the second power-drum reading for the focused triple lines, and record this figure as the minus-cylinder power of the lens.

6. Read the axis of the cylinder off the cylinder axis wheel.

Measuring Bifocal Power

1. After measuring the sphere and cylinder distance portion of bifocal eyeglass lenses, center the bifocal add at the bottom of the lens in the lensmeter **gimbal** (the ring like frame) and refocus on the single lines.

2. The add, or bifocal reading, is the algebraic difference between the distance reading of the single line focus and the new single line focus.

3. Always read from the same type of line (single) in the distance part and the bifocal part to determine the bifocal strength.

4. When measuring the add power in progressive addition lenses, take care to select the area with the least distortion in both the distance and the reading portions of the lenses before taking a reading. Be sure to read the add as close to the bottom of the lens as possible.

5. Because the add power is on the front surface of the lens, to accurately measure add powers over 2.50, the lenses need to be flipped over so that the temples faced towards you. For higher add powers, reading the power from the back surface of the lens will overestimate the add strength.

Measuring Prism Power and Orientation

In general, the existence of prescribed prism power in an eyeglass lens is revealed when the lensometer mires cannot be centered in the central portion of the lensometer target. Once you have determined the presence of a prism, measure prism power and determine orientation as follows:

1. Count the number of black concentric circles from the central cross of the lensometer target to the center of the vertical and/or horizontal crossed mires. Each circle represents one prism diopter.

2. Record the base direction of the prism by determining the direction of the displacement of the mires. For example, if the mires are displaced upward, the prism base is up; downward displacement indicates base down; displacement towards the nose, base in; and displacement towards the temple, base out.

3. Auxiliary prisms may be needed to assist in measuring glasses with prism power greater than the number of concentric circles.

4. To accurately determine vertical prism measurements, center the highest powered lens first. Without moving the table, switch to the lower powered lens and record the prism amount and direction.

5. For horizontal prism, mark the patient's interpupillary distance on their spectacles. Then check the prism power and direction when measuring through the spot where the patient's pupils line up on the spectacles.

c. Direct ophthalmoscope

The direct ophthalmoscope works by illuminating the patient's fundus. In doing this, light reflecting off the patient's retina is refracted by their lens and cornea, causing the light rays to leave the patient's eye parallel, if the patient is emmetropic. If the patient is myopic, the light rays leaving the patient's eyes are converging, requiring the use of a minus lens in the ophthalmoscope for the observer to see the retina clearly. If the patient is hyperopic, the light rays leaving the patient's eyes are diverging, requiring the use of a plus lens in the ophthalmoscope for the observer to see the retina clearly. The direct ophthalmoscope has auxiliary lenses built into it to correct for any refractive error the patient or the observer might have.

With the direct ophthalmoscope, the image of the retina is upright. Magnification is based on the total refractive power of the eye. Using the basic magnification formula of $M = F/4$, an emmetropic eye of +60.00D would provide $+60/4 = +15X$. An aphakic eye of +40.00D would provide $+40/4 = +10X$.

d. Indirect Ophthalmoscopy

Indirect ophthalmoscopy works on the principle of an astronomical telescope, where the patient's cornea and lens act as the telescopes objective lens and the condensing lens acts as the telescopes eyepiece lens. Because indirect ophthalmoscopy uses two plus lenses in a telescopic arrangement, the fundus is the object of the condensing lens. The image formed by this system is located above the condensing lens and is called an aerial image. This image of the fundus is larger and inverted.

The two plus lenses (the eye and the condensing lens) determine the magnification of the aerial image. For the emmetropic eye, using the formula $M_A = (-)D_{Eye}/C_{condensing\ lens} = (-)60/D$ (condensing lens), we find that a 20D condensing lens results in $(-)60/20 = -3X$.

As the power of the condensing lens decreases, the magnification increases. Axial magnification increases exponentially, based on the formula *Axial magnification*:
$$M_A = (M)^2$$

e. Keratometer

The keratometer is an instrument that uses the reflecting power of the cornea to measure its curvature/refractive power. This is accomplished by measuring the radius of curvature of the central 3mm of the cornea. The central cornea can be thought of as a high powered (~250D) convex spherical mirror. The formula used to determine the curvature/refractive power of the cornea is: $D = (n-1)/r$. Where D is the reflecting power of the cornea, n is the standardize refractive index of the cornea (1.3375) and r is the radius of curvature of the central cornea.

To determine the radius of curvature of the cornea (r), keratometers employ the relationship that exist between the object and image size of a convex mirror. Keratometers determine r by either varying the image size to a get a known object size, or by varying the object size to get a known image size. Keratometers use optical doubling (page ??) prisms to allow for the measurement of the unknown size.

When computing the anticipated astigmatic correction based on the keratometry readings, the clinician takes the amount of with the rule astigmatism noted by the keratometry readings, multiply that by 1.25 and then subtract that number from 0.75 diopters (lenticular astigmatism). For example, if an individual has 1.00 diopter of with the rule corneal astigmatism, the expected refractive astigmatism is calculated as follows; 1.00D x 1.25 - 0.75D = 1.25D - 0.75D = 0.50D

f. Gonioscope

Total Internal Reflection (TIR) makes it impossible to view the anterior chamber angle without the use of a gonioscopic contact lens. Normally light from the angle undergoes TIR at the air-tear film interface. As result of this, the light from the angle is not able to escape from the eye making the angle impossible to visualize. This problem is overcome by the gonioscopic contact lens which sits on the cornea. In this way, the air at the surface of the cornea is eliminated. Total internal reflection occurs when light is trapped in the incident medium. Because TIR never occurs when light travels from a lower to a higher index, light is able to enter the gonioscopic contact lens where it is reflected by the gonioscopic mirror. This allows the angle of the anterior chamber to be visualized by the examiner.

Gonioscopic tilt angle should be approximately 7.5 degrees to the visual axis. This minimizes reflections and image distortion.

g. Retinoscope/Retinoscopy

History of Retinoscopy

The technique of retinoscopy was first introduced by Cuignet in 1873. Initially, retinoscopes were illuminated externally with candles, sunlight, lamps, or bulbs from which the light was captured with a mirror. The earliest retinoscope designs were spot retinoscopes. In the 1920s, Jack Copeland patented the first streak retinoscope.

Retinoscopy

A technique that allows the clinician to objectively determine the spherical power and the cylinder power and axis (both regular and irregular). Because retinoscopy is an objective test, it frees the clinician from dependence on patient responses. This allows the clinician to determine the refractive state of pre-verbal and non-verbal patients of all ages. Additionally, retinoscopy allows the clinician to visualize anterior segment opacities or optical irregularities.

Most retinoscope today use a streak projection system. This streak of light is reflected from a mirror. Additionally, the streak can be moved in relation to a convex lens in the device by way of the sleeve. This allows the light to leave the device as if it were coming from a point behind the retinoscope (plano mirror setting) or as if it were coming from a point between the examiner and the patient (concave mirror setting). For Copeland retinoscopes, the plano position is with the sleeve up, while the Welch Allyn (and all others) retinoscope is in the plano position with the sleeve down.

Retinoscopy may be performed under static (accommodation is at rest or paralyzed) or dynamic (accommodation is active) conditions.

Normally, the examiner will use their right eye to perform retinoscopy on the patient's right eye and their left eye for the patient's left eye. The examiner should align themselves just off-center to minimize lens reflections and to allow the patient to visualize the distance target to relax their accommodation. The patient should be instructed to look at a distance target such as a large Snellen letter (20/200-20/400), therefore putting the patient's accommodation at rest.

When performing retinoscopy, the clinician shines the beam of the scope into the patient's pupil in order to see the retinal reflex. The beam is perpendicular to the meridian being scoped. This means that when the beam is oriented vertically and moved side to side, it is moving along the horizontal meridian and thus measuring power in the horizontal meridian. When the beam is oriented horizontally and moved up and down, it is moving along the vertical meridian and thus measuring power in the vertical meridian.

- When doing retinoscopy, the examiner is attempting to put the far point of the patient's eye at the plane of the examiner's pupil.
  - When the reflex shows "against" motion, the far point plane lies between the patient's eye and the examiner's eye, indicating myopia.
  - When the reflex shows "with" motion, the far point lies outside the interval between the patient's eye and the observer's eye, indicating hyperopia, emmetropia or mild myopia.

The endpoint of retinoscopy is neutrality. Neutrality is reached when the clinician sees a bright, broad, fast reflex. There are three main characteristics tell the clinician about their proximity to neutrality:

- Speed: the faster the reflex, the closer to neutral
- Brilliance: the brighter, more brilliant the reflex, the closer to neutral
- Width: the broader the reflex, the closer to neutral

There are varying opinions about when neutrality is reached. Some feel the first "against motion" coming from "with motion" is neutrality. Others the last "with motion". Rarely will there be a precise neutral point. The key is for the clinician to be consistent in establishing neutrality. This will allow for a predictable amount of "clinician error".

Clinician Error occurs when the clinician;

- Does not control the patient's accommodation
- Does not maintain their working distance
- Overshoots or undershoots neutrality

Question: If you obtain "with motion" during retinoscopy, is the far point of the patient in front of the peep hole, at the peep hole, or beyond the peep hole?

Answer: Beyond the peephole. The goal of neutralization is to have the light reflex of the patient's far point at the peephole. The light at the patient's pupil fills the entire space at once when neutrality is reached. "With" motion requires more plus to be added to the prescription to move the far point to neutralization. "Against" motion means that the far point is in front of the peephole. Therefore, more minus must be added to move the far point to neutralization.

See page 103 for a full description of how to perform retinoscopy when doing a plus cylinder refraction. See page 108 for minus cylinder refractions.

h: Optical Doubling

Optical doubling is the technique used in pachymetry, keratometry and applanation tonometry to allow these instruments to make their respective measurements. Optical doubling uses two prisms placed base to base. This creates two images for the clinician to view that are separated by a fixed amount.

In **Goldman tonometry**, the applanation head is exactly 3.06 mm in size. The optical doubling prism incorporated into the applanation head creates two images that are offset by 3.06 mm when the proper amount of pressure is applied to the cornea.

i. Handheld Lenses for Slit Lamp Microscopy

Hand lenses used during slit lamp microscopy are designed to either nullify the high refractive power of the cornea, or use the power of the cornea as a component of an astronomical telescope, similar to what is done with indirect ophthalmoscopy. In all cases, the imaged formed by these lenses is formed within the focal range of the slit lamp microscope. Without these lenses, the clinician would not be able to visualize the retina with the slit lamp microscope.

Goldmann contact lenses and other lenses of similar design nullify the cornea refractive power. By placing these lenses on the cornea, a virtual and erect image of the retina is created near the pupillary plane.

A Hruby lens is a -58.6D plano-concave lens that is held just in front of the cornea. This lens creates a virtual and erect image of the retina near the pupillary plane.

High powered biconvex condensing lenses (60D, 78D and 90D) use the same optical principle as indirect ophthalmoscopy. These lenses create an inverted, real image in front of the lens.

j. A-Scan

A-scan biometry is a device that uses sound waves in the 8-15 MHz range to produce a display of reflectivity versus time for the single direction the A-scan probe is pointing. This tool is used to calculate intraocular lens power, measure extraocular muscle thickness as well as measure intraocular tumor heights.

k. Bagolini Lenses

Bagolini lenses are Plano lenses that have tiny striations (0.005 mm in width) inscribed into them. These lenses are used to test for normal retinal correspondence (NRC) versus anomalous retinal correspondence (ARC), versus absent binocular vision. To test with these lenses, the lenses are oriented before each eye of the patient with the axis of striations at an angle 90° apart. For example, the striations might be placed at 45° for the right eye and 135° for the left eye. The test is performed both at distance (20 feet or 6 meters) and at near (13 inches or 33 centimeters). With the lenses in place, a small fixation light is viewed through the lenses. This creates a weak luminance ray oriented perpendicular to the striations on the glass, similar to the effect produced by a Maddox lens. If suppression is present, only one oblique line corresponding to that seen by the non-suppressing eye is visualized. The advantage of this test is that the patient views through a more normal visual environment, in contrast to the Worth 4-Dot test.

l. Duochrome (Red-Green) Test

See pages 86, 107, and 111 for a description of the Duochrome test and how it is used clinically.

m. Worth 4-Dot

The Worth 4-Dot test is a simple test for fusion, suppression and anomalous retinal correspondence. Testing can be done at any distance. For this testing, the patient wears a red filter before one eye and a green filter before the other. They are then exposed to four lights: two green, one red and one white. Normal individuals will see the white light through both filters, the green lights are seen through only the green filter and the red light is seen only through the red filter. Patients with fusion report that there are four lights, but the white light is a fluctuating mixture of red and green due to color rivalry.

n. Stereo Fly Test

Stereopsis testing is performed with the Stereo Fly Test. The Stereo Fly test allows for the testing of both gross and fine stereo vision. Stereopsis is quantified into the seconds of arc of retinal image disparity required to produce the perception of 3 dimensions. Stereopsis testing is designed to determine the minimum disparity needed to elicit a response. For very minimal quantities of retinal image disparity to be appreciated, the images must simultaneously project onto the retinal area having maximum resolving power. Maximum resolving power occurs within the maculas. Extra macular single binocular vision provides gross stereopsis but fine stereopsis is a product of macular binocular vision.

Fine stereopsis is a product of macular binocular vision. Individuals without macular binocular vision have an average stereo acuity of 200 seconds of arc and never better than 67 seconds of arc. The average person with macular binocular vision has an average stereo acuity of 24 seconds of arc and possibly as good as 14 seconds of arc.

lower seconds of arc ↑ (better) stereo

40. Miscellaneous Information

a. LensTilt

The position of the optical center will vary with the tilt of the lens before the eyes. The ideal tilt of standard lenses is 8 degrees in on the bottom of the lens. Such a tilt places the optical center 4mm below the center of the pupil when the line of sight passes normally through the lens surface.

When the lens is tilted, the incident light strikes the lens obliquely, inducing marginal or radial astigmatism even though the light passes through the center of the lens.

The change in power of the sphere through tilting is determined by the formula: $F(1 + 1/3 \sin^2 a)$. The created cylinder power is determined by the formula: $F(\tan^2 a)$, where a = the angle of tilt.

If a cylinder lens is tilted on its axis, no actual sphere power is induced however the total new cylinder power is increased by the formula previously noted.

The effect of tilting a minus spherical lens is the production of minus cylinder at the axis of rotation – 180 degrees. The cylinder power increases with both the degree of the tilt and the power of the lens.

A simplified formula to determine the change in sphere power is to take $(1/10$ the amount of tilt$)^2$ = the percentage of power added to the original sphere. The increase in the cylindrical correct is approximately equal to 3x the induced sphere increase.

Examples of simplified formula:

A +3.00D sphere tilted 20 degrees will result in what spherical power increase? – $(20/10)^2 = 4\%$, .04 x 3.00D = 0.12D

A +3.00D sphere tilted 20 degrees will result in a compound effect of +3.12 combined with +0.40 cylinder. Simplified formula – $(20/10)^2 = 4\%$, .04 x 3.00D = 0.12D

A +1.00D sphere tilted 45 degrees will result in a compound effect of +1.16, combined with +1.00 cylinder.

An under corrected myope will therefore be able to obtain better distance acuity by tilting his glasses. For example, the effect of tilting a –10.00 diopter lens 10 degrees along the horizontal axis results in an optical correction of –10.10 –0.31 x 180 which gives a spherical equivalent of –10.25D. If the same lens is tilted 30 degrees, the resultant effective optical correction is −10.83 −3.33 x 180 with a spherical equivalent of −12.50 diopters. This is why an under-corrected myope tilts their spectacles to attain better distance vision.

Question: A point source is placed 50 cm from a cylindrical lens of +5.00 diopters, axis 90 degrees. Find the position and direction of the line foci formed by this lens.

Answer: Do this yourself to understand how this works.

b. Pinhole Visual Acuity

For individuals who do not have any type of ocular disease, a pinhole aperture can be a useful tool in determining if a refractive error is present or if a refractive change is needed. The most useful pinhole diameter for clinical purposes is 1.2 millimeters. This size pinhole will be effective for refractive errors of +/− 5.00D. A pinhole improves visual acuity by decreasing the size of the blur circle on the retina resulting in an improvement of the individual's visual acuity. However, if the pinhole aperture is smaller than 1.2 millimeters, the blurring effects of diffraction around the edges of the aperture will actually increase the blur circle, causing the vision to be worse.

Individuals with macular disease, as well as other ocular diseases that affect central vision, may have similar or even reduced acuity when looking through a pinhole. This is because the reduced amount of light entering through the pinhole makes the chart less clear. Additionally, it can be difficult to use eccentric fixation through a pinhole. For this reason, individuals with ocular disease should not be told that a spectacle correction change will not improve their vision, based solely on their looking through a pinhole. Careful retinoscopy along with a trial frame refraction is needed to determine whether an individual with pathology induced vision loss will benefit from a spectacle correction change.

c. Standard Subjective Refraction with Plus Cylinder Photopter

Prior to starting your refraction, baseline visual acuities (OD, OS and OU) must be determined. Accurately assessing visual acuity is important for many reasons. It allows the clinician to:

- Determine best corrected acuity with refraction
- Monitor the effect of treatment and/or progression of disease

- Estimate the dioptric power of optical devices necessary for reading regular size print
- Verify eligibility for tasks such as driving
- Verify eligibility as "legally blind"

Plus cylinder phoropter

The goal of the subjective refraction is to achieve clear and comfortable binocular vision. The ability of the clinician to maintain control during the refraction is directly related to their ability to communicate clearly and directly with the patient.

Set up

- Before putting the phoropter in front of the patient, clear the phoropter, set the cylinder axis at 90 degrees and unocclude both eyes.
- After positioning the phoropter in front of the patient, level the phoropter and make sure the interpupillary distance is properly adjusted.
- Put a non-accommodative target (20/200 or 20/400 letter) on the chart.

Retinoscopy

- Start with a horizontally oriented, plano mirror streak (sleeve up on Copeland and sleeve down on Welch-Allyn) to streak the vertical meridian.
- Neutralize this meridian by adding plus lenses for 'with motion' or minus lenses for 'against motion'.
- Once neutralized, rotate your streak 90 degrees.
- Now with a vertically oriented streak, streak the horizontal meridian.
- If your patient has no astigmatism, there will be no motion. Retinoscopy is completed for this eye.
- If your patient has 'with the rule' astigmatism, you will see 'with motion' which you will neutralize by adding plus cylinder axis 90.
- If your patient has 'against the rule' astigmatism, you will see 'against motion'. If 'against motion' is noted, you will neutralize this by adding minus spherical power.
- For 'against the rule' astigmatism, after neutralizing the horizontal meridian with sphere power, rotate the cylinder axis on the phoropter to 180 degrees. Next, rotate your streak back to the horizontal meridian. You should now see 'with motion' in the vertical meridian that you will neutralize by adding plus cylinder axis 180.
- Once you have neutralized the right eye, do the same for the left eye.

- When you have neutralized both eyes by retinoscopy, remove your working distance lens from each eye (1.50D for a 66 centimeter working distance or 2.00D for a 50 centimeter working distance).

Initial Maximum Plus to Maximum Visual Acuity (MPMVA)

- Next, occlude the left eye, put several lines of letters on the eye chart (20/20 – 20/30 or 20/20-20/40) and ask the patient to read the smallest line they can.
- Assuming the patient can read the letters being presented; begin adding +0.25D steps to the phoropter until the patient has lost 2 lines of vision.
- Next, slowly decrease the power in the phoropter (less plus or more minus), in 0.25D steps, until the patient is able to see the 20/20 line or until there is no further improvement in vision. Expect about a one line improvement on the eye chart for every –0.25D added.
- Once you have achieved the initial maximum plus to maximum visual acuity, the patient's cylindrical correction can be refined.

Refining Cylinder Axis and Power

- Swing the Jackson Cross Cylinder (JCC) in front of the patient's eye to check for cylinder axis and power.
- As a general rule, if the patient's refractive error is primarily cylindrical, or if by retinoscopy you found more then 1.00D of cylinder, start by checking the cylinder axis first. Otherwise, start by checking the cylinder power.
- To check cylinder power, adjust the position of the JCC so that the white or red dots correspond with the cylinder axis.
- With the patient looking at a single line of letters, one line larger than their best visual acuity found during the initial MPMVA…
- Tell the patient, "I am going to give you two choice, neither choice will be perfectly clear, however, I want you to tell me, which lens choice is clearer; choice one or choice two; choice three or choice four, etc.?"
- If the patient chooses the white dot, add +0.50D of cylindrical power while remembering to add –0.25D of spherical power (to maintain spherical equivalent).
- If the patient chooses the red dot, remove +0.50D of cylindrical power and add +0.25D of spherical power(to maintain spherical equivalent).
- Once the patient reverses; chooses the red dot after previously choosing the white or vice versa, adjust the cylinder power by 0.25D in the opposite direction of your

previous change. The spherical power does not need to be adjusted for this 0.25D change.

- Once again, check the cylindrical power with the JCC to see if the patient wants more or less power. The goal is to give the least amount of cylindrical power that provides the clearest vision.

- When you have completed checking the cylinder power, you next check the cylinder axis by positioning the JCC so that the white and red dots straddle (45 degrees on either side) the cylindrical axis.

- Again ask the patient, which lens choice is clearer, choice one or choice two, etc.?

- Move the axis in the direction of the white dot, initially in 15 degree increments, decreasing the increments size, following a reversal (15 to 10 to 5 to 3 to 1 degree) as the axis is refined.

- Once the cylindrical power and axis have been refined with the JCC, remove the JCC from in front of the patient's eye and ask the patient to read the smallest line they can.

Cylinder Power Search

- If retinoscopy and lensometry suggest no cylinder is needed and you suspect there may be some, do a cylinder power search.

- With your JCC oriented for power at 90 and 180 degrees, ask the patient which is better, choice one or two.

- If no preference, repeat at 45 and 135 degrees.

- If the patient has a preference, add +0.50 cylinder at the axis of preference, along with –0.25D sphere.

- Using standard JCC technique described above, refine the cylinder power and axis.

Second Maximum Plus to Maximum Visual Acuity (MPMVA)

- Again, begin adding +0.25D steps to the phoropter until the patient has lost 2 lines of vision.

- Next, slowly decrease the power in the phoropter (less plus or more minus), in 0.25D steps, until the patient is able to see the 20/20 line or until there is no further improvement in vision.

- Occlude the right eye while unoccluding the left. Repeat the same process for the left eye, beginning with the Initial Maximum Plus to Maximum Visual Acuity.

- Special Note: Experienced refractionists typically skip this step because they are reasonably sure they have not over-minused the patient by this point. Beginning refractionists should not skip this step until they have done their first 1,000 refractions.

Binocular Balance

- Once the monocular subjective refraction has been completed, it is time for the binocular balance. Binocular balancing is only done when the visual acuity is relatively equal between the two eyes.

- Binocular balancing can be accomplished in two different ways. Binocular balancing can be done using the Risley prism on the phoropter or by alternate occlusion. In either case, you should start the binocular balancing procedures by adding +0.50 to +0.75D sphere to both eyes so that the patient's visual acuity is blurred to the 20/30 – 20/40 level. By slightly blurring vision in this way, eye dominance is effectively neutralized during the balancing process.

Risley Prism Binocular Balancing Technique

- Using the Risley prisms, applied 3 prism diopters base up in front of the right eye and 3 prism diopters based down in front of the left eye. This will result in the right eye seeing the lower image and the left eye seeing the upper image.

- Asking the patient to ignore brightness differences (this can be confusing for some patients), have them tell you which image appears clearer. Add +0.25D to the clearer eye to fog it further.

- Again ask the patient which image is clearer, add +0.25D to the clearer eye.

- The end point is reached when either both sets of letters look the same, or when the patient's dominant eye appears slightly clearer than their non-dominant eye.

Alternate Occlusion Technique

- After fogging the patient, alternately cover one eye and then the other eye while asking the patient which eye sees the chart more clearly; eye one or eye two (to avoid confusion, say "eye one" or "eye two" not "right eye" or "left eye" as you alternately occlude). Add +0.25D to the clearer eye to fog it further.

- The end point is reached when either both sets of letters look the same, or when the patient's dominant eye appears slightly clearer than their non-dominant eye.

Determining the Final Correction

- Once the binocular balance is completed, add –0.25D OU, one step at a time to bring the patient back to their best visual acuity. Remember, you should expect about one line of improvement in vision with each –0.25D you add.

- Do not give additional minus spherical power without an improvement in acuity.

Duochrome Test

- Duochrome (red-green) test - can be used as a monocular or binocular test to determine the proper spherical power. With this test, if the letters on the green side of the chart appear blacker, add +0.25D. If the letters on the red side of the chart appear blacker, add –0.25D. The endpoint is reached when the letters appear equally black on both the red and green side. It is important to ask the patient to tell you which side the letters look "blacker" on, not which side they look "clearer" on.

Cardinal Rules of Refraction

- Keep It Simple - keep the description of what you are doing as simple as possible.
- Maintain Your Patience - go slowly when needed and try to make the choices as easy as possible to avoid frustration by both you and your patient.
- Provide Encouragement - particularly when working with patients that are hard to refract.
- Proceed with a Purpose - do not offer more choices than are necessary to establish your endpoint. Boredom and fatigue can result in poor subjective responses.

Our ultimate goal is to make both images looked the same, yet we continually are asking which is better, knowing that the decision gets harder as we get closer to our goal of equality.

Favorite Phrases

- During the subjective portion of the refraction say – "I am going to have you look through two different lenses. Although neither lens may be perfect, I want you to tell me which one looks clearer".
- When the patient becomes indecisive, remember to add - "or do they look the same?" Advise them it is OK to think the choices look about the same.

d. Standard Subjective Refraction with Minus Cylinder Photopter

The goal of the subjective refraction is to achieve clear and comfortable binocular vision. The ability of the clinician to maintain control during the refraction is directly related to their ability to communicate clearly and directly with the patient.

Set up

- Before putting the phoropter in front of the patient, clear the phoropter, set the cylinder axis at 180 degrees and unocclude both eyes.
- After positioning the phoropter in front of the patient, level the phoropter and make sure the interpupillary distance is properly adjusted.
- Put a non-accommodative target (20/200 or 20/400 letter) on the chart.

Retinoscopy

- Start with a vertically oriented, plano mirror streak (sleeve up on Copeland and sleeve down on Welch-Allyn) to streak the horizontal meridian.
- Neutralize this meridian by adding plus lenses for 'with motion' or minus lenses for 'against motion'.
- Once neutralized, rotate your streak 90 degrees.
- Now with a horizontally oriented streak, streak the vertical meridian.
- If your patient has no astigmatism, there will be no motion. Retinoscopy is completed for this eye.
- If your patient has 'with the rule' astigmatism, you will see 'against motion' which you will neutralize by adding minus cylinder axis 180.
- If your patient has 'against the rule' astigmatism, you will see 'against motion'. If 'against motion' is noted, you will neutralize this by adding minus spherical power.
- For 'against the rule' astigmatism, after neutralizing the vertical meridian with sphere power, rotate the cylinder axis on the phoropter to 90 degrees. Next, rotate your streak back to the vertical meridian. You should now see 'against motion' in the horizontal meridian that you will neutralize by adding minus cylinder axis 90.
- Once you have neutralized the right eye, do the same for the left eye.
- When you have neutralized both eyes by retinoscopy, remove your working distance lens from each eye (1.50D for a 66 centimeter working distance or 2.00D for a 50 centimeter working distance).

Initial Maximum Plus to Maximum Visual Acuity (MPMVA)

- Next, occlude the left eye, put several lines of letters on the eye chart (20/20 – 20/30 or 20/20-20/40) and ask the patient to read the smallest line they can.
- Assuming the patient can read the letters being presented; begin adding +0.25D steps to the phoropter until the patient has lost 2 lines of vision.
- Next, slowly decrease the power in the phoropter (less plus or more minus), in 0.25D steps, until the patient is able to see the 20/20 line or until there is no further

improvement in vision. Expect about a one line improvement on the eye chart for every -0.25D added.

- Once you have achieve the initial maximum plus to maximum visual acuity, the patient's cylindrical correction can be refined.

Refining Cylinder Axis and Power

- Swing the Jackson Cross Cylinder (JCC) in front of the patient's eye to check for cylinder axis and power.
- As a general rule, if the patient's refractive error is primarily cylindrical, or if by retinoscopy you found more then 1.00D of cylinder, start by checking the cylinder axis first. Otherwise, start by checking the cylinder power.
- To check cylinder power, adjust the position of the JCC so that the white or red dots correspond with the cylinder axis.
- With the patient looking at a single line of letters, one line larger than their best visual acuity found during the initial MPMVA…
- Tell the patient, "I am going to give you two choice, neither choice will be perfectly clear, however, I want you to tell me, which lens choice is clearer; choice one or choice two; choice three or choice four, etc.?"
- Be sure to use fresh choices and new numbers with each pair of choices presented.
- If the patient chooses the white dot, subtract -0.50D of cylindrical power while remembering to add -0.25D of spherical power (to maintain spherical equivalent).
- If the patient chooses the red dot, add -0.50D of cylindrical power and add +0.25D of spherical power(to maintain spherical equivalent).
- Once the patient reverses; chooses the red dot after previously choosing the white or vice versa, adjust the cylinder power by 0.25D in the opposite direction of your previous change. The spherical power does not need to be adjusted for this 0.25D change.
- Once again, check the cylindrical power with the JCC to see if the patient wants more or less power. The goal is to give the least amount of cylindrical power that provides the clearest vision.
- When you have completed checking the cylinder power, you next check the cylinder axis by positioning the JCC so that the white and red dots straddle (45 degrees on either side) the cylindrical axis.
- Again ask the patient, which lens choice is clearer, choice one or choice two, etc.?

- Move the axis in the direction of the white dot, initially in 15 degree increments, decreasing the increments size, following a reversal (15 to 10 to 5 to 3 to 1 degree) as the axis is refined.
- Once the cylindrical power and axis have been refined with the JCC, remove the JCC from in front of the patient's eye and ask the patient to read the smallest line they can.

Cylinder Power Search

- If retinoscopy and lensometry suggest no cylinder is needed and you suspect there may be some, do a cylinder power search.
- With your JCC oriented for power at 90 and 180 degrees, ask the patient which is better, choice one or two.
- If no preference, repeat at 45 and 135 degrees.
- If the patient has a preference, add -0.50 cylinder at the axis of preference, along with +0.25D sphere.
- Using standard JCC technique described above, refine the cylinder power and axis.

Second Maximum Plus to Maximum Visual Acuity (MPMVA)

- Again, begin adding +0.25D steps to the phoropter until the patient has lost 2 lines of vision.
- Next, slowly decrease the power in the phoropter (less plus or more minus), in 0.25D steps, until the patient is able to see the 20/20 line or until there is no further improvement in vision.
- Occlude the right eye while unoccluding the left. Repeat the same process for the left eye, beginning with the Initial Maximum Plus to Maximum Visual Acuity.
- Special Note: Experienced refractionists typically skip this step because they are reasonably sure they have not over-minused the patient by this point. Beginning refractionists should not skip this step until they have done their first 1,000 refractions.

Binocular Balance

- Once the monocular subjective refraction has been completed, it is time for the binocular balance. Binocular balancing is only done when the visual acuity is relatively equal between the two eyes.
- Binocular balancing can be accomplished in two different ways. Binocular balancing can be done using the Risley prism on the phoropter or by alternate

occlusion. In either case, you should start the binocular balancing procedures by adding +0.50 to +0.75D sphere to both eyes so that the patient's visual acuity is blurred to the 20/30 – 20/40 level. By slightly blurring vision in this way, eye dominance is effectively neutralized during the balancing process.

Risley Prism Binocular Balancing Technique

▪ Using the Risley prisms, applied 3 prism diopters base up in front of the right eye and 3 prism diopters based down in front of the left eye. This will result in the right eye seeing the lower image and the left eye seeing the upper image.

▪ Asking the patient to ignore brightness differences (this can be confusing for some patients), have them tell you which image appears clearer. Add +0.25D to the clearer eye to fog it further.

▪ Again ask the patient which image is clearer, add +0.25D to the clearer eye.

▪ The end point is reached when either both sets of letters look the same, or when the patient's dominant eye appears slightly clearer than their non-dominant eye.

Alternate Occlusion Technique

▪ After fogging the patient, alternately cover one eye and then the other eye while asking the patient which eye sees the chart more clearly; eye one or eye two (to avoid confusion, say "eye one" or "eye two" not "right eye" or "left eye" as you alternately occlude). Add +0.25D to the clearer eye to fog it further.

▪ The end point is reached when either both sets of letters look the same, or when the patient's dominant eye appears slightly clearer than their non-dominant eye.

Determining the Final Correction

▪ Once the binocular balance is completed, add -0.25D OU, one step at a time to bring the patient back to their best visual acuity. Remember, you should expect about one line of improvement in vision with each -0.25D you add.

▪ Do not give additional minus spherical power without an improvement in acuity.

Duochrome Test

▪ Duochrome (red - green) test - can be used as a monocular or binocular test to determine the proper spherical power. With this test, if the letters on the green side of the chart appear blacker, add +0.25D. If the letters on the red side of the chart appear blacker, add -0.25D. The endpoint is reached when the letters appear equally black on both the red and green side. It is important to ask the patient to tell you which side the letters look "blacker" on, not which side they look "clearer" on.

e. Optical Cross

All spectacle corrections can be broken down to their component powers by putting them on an optical cross. It is important to remember that the cylindrical power is always oriented 90 degrees from the cylinder axis. For example, the prescription +2.00 +1.00 x 090 is drawn as follows:

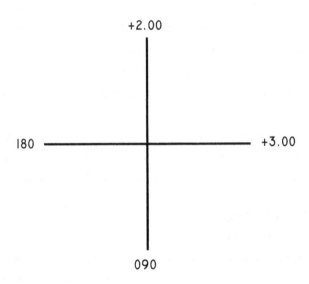

The optical cross can be useful when doing retinoscopy with loose lenses or a retinoscopy bar. For example, when doing retinoscopy at a 67 cm working distance, the vertical meridian (horizontal streak) is neutralized with a +0.50D lens. The horizontal meridian (vertical streak) is neutralized with a +1.50D lens. The gross retinoscopy findings are drawn on an optical cross as follows.

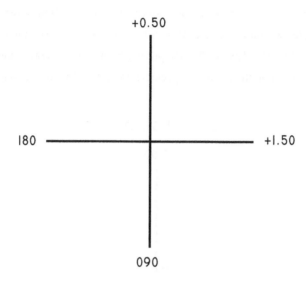

Next, the working distance lens must be removed from both meridians. The working distance lens for 67 cm is 100/67 = 1.50D. The optical cross powers are adjusted as follows.

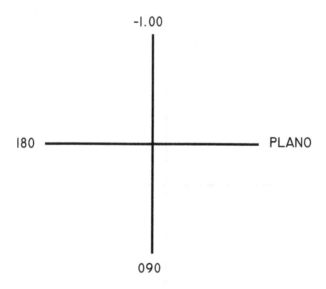

The spectacle correction for this optical cross is written as −1.00 +1.00 x 090 in plus cylinder or Plano −1.00 x 180 in minus cylinder.

Another use for the optical cross is when doing an over refraction. Example, a patient is wearing spectacles with a correction of –3.00 +1.50 x 080. By retinoscopy, you find an over refraction of +0.50 +1.00 x 170. By putting both of these corrections on an optical cross, you can determine the resultant spectacle correction by combining the two powers for each meridian.

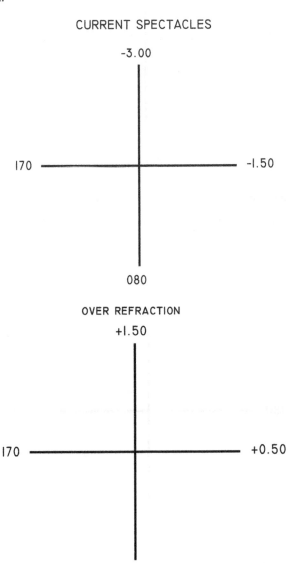

CURRENT SPECTACLES

-3.00

170 ————————————— -1.50

080

OVER REFRACTION

+1.50

170 ————————————— +0.50

080

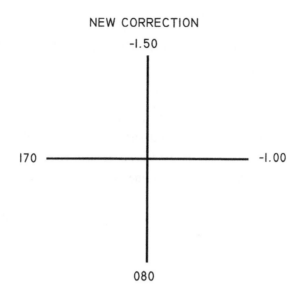

NEW CORRECTION

The new spectacle correction is −1.50 +0.50 x 080 in plus cylinder and −1.00−0.50 x 170 in minus cylinder.

f. Prescribing Glasses

Question: What do you check when a patient complains that their new glasses are not as good as their previous pair?

Answer:

1. Ask specifically what the complaint is. Distance? Near? Asthenopia? Diplopia? Pain behind the ears or at the bridge of the nose from ill fitting glasses?
2. Read the new and old glasses on the lensometer and compare. Make sure the old glasses did not have any prism. Check the patient for undetected strabismus with cover testing.
3. Refract the patient again. Possibly, with a cycloplegic agent, if the symptoms warrant.
4. Check the optical centers in comparison with the pupillary centers.
5. Check whether the reading segments are in the correct position—level with the lower lid.
6. Make sure the new glasses fit the patient correctly.
7. Check whether the old glasses were made with a plus cylinder using the Geneva lens clock.
8. Check whether the base curve has changed with the Geneva lens clock.
9. Evaluate the patient for dry eyes.
10. If the patient has a high prescription, check the vertex distance. Often is it easier to refract such patients over their old pair of glasses to keep the same vertex distance.
11. Check the pantoscopic tilt. Normally the tilt is 10-15 degrees so that when the patient reads, the eye is perpendicular to the lens. If the tilt is off, especially in relation to the old glasses, the patient may notice.
12. With postoperative glasses, evaluate for diplopia in downgaze due to anisometropia.
13. Perhaps the add is too strong or too weak. Check the patient using trial lenses and reading material.
14. Sometimes if the diameter of the lens is much larger in the newer frame, the patient may be noticing distortion in the periphery of their lenses. In this situation, encourage a smaller frame. Conversely, if the new frame is significantly smaller, the patient may notice the edges of the lenses or, the reading area of their multifocal lens may be too small to use efficiently. In this situation, encourage a larger frame.
15. Above all, try to test the new prescription in a trial frame with a walk around the office; you do not want to go through this process again.

g. *Trial Frame/Low Vision Refraction*

Prior to starting your refraction, baseline visual acuities (OD, OS and OU) must be determined. Accurately assessing visual acuity is important for many reasons. It allows the clinician to:

- Determine best corrected acuity with refraction
- Monitor the effect of treatment and/or progression of disease
- Estimate the dioptric power of optical devices necessary for reading regular size print
- Verify eligibility for tasks such as driving
- Verify eligibility as "legally blind"

Trial Frame Refraction Techniques

The goal of the subjective refraction is to achieve clear and comfortable (binocular, if possible) vision.

The ability of the clinician to maintain control during the refraction is directly related to their ability to communicate clearly and directly with the patient.

Disadvantages of a Phoropter

- The light reflex for retinoscopy is poorer than with loose lenses
- There is decreased light transmission when multiple lenses are used
- Eccentric viewing is difficult to impossible with a phoropter
- It is difficult for the patient to use their null point (nystagmus) with a phoropter
- It is difficult to use Just Noticeable Difference (JND) refraction techniques with a phoropter.

Trial Frame Refraction

- A trial frame and loose lenses are easier and more natural than a phoropter for patients that are difficult to refract or those that are visually impaired.
- Standard refraction techniques are employed when performing a trial frame refraction on an individual with normal sight.
- Just Noticeable Difference refraction techniques are used for individuals that are visually impaired.
- When in doubt, use the trial frame.

Just Noticeable Difference (JND) Refraction Techniques

- JND is the amount of lens power needed to elicit an appreciable change in clarity or blur
- The poorer the visual acuity, the larger the JND
- JND equals the denominator of the 20 foot Snellen acuity/100
- Example: 20/150: 150/100 = 1.50D. Start with +/–0.75D
- JND allows accurate refraction at any acuity level
- JND refracting techniques apply to both sphere and cylinder corrections
- JND elicits reliable answers

Case Example: JND Sphere

- VA sc: 20/400, no old spectacles and unable to do retinoscopy
- 400/100 = 4.00D. Start with +/–2.00D
- Patient states +2.00D is clearer. Put +4.00D in the trial frame
- With +4.00D in the trial frame, again asked the patient to compare +2.00D/–2.00D. If the patient still prefers +2.00D, replace the +4.00D lens in the trial frame with a +8.00D lens.
- With +8.00D in the trial frame, again asked the patient to compare +2.00D/–2.00D. If the patient now prefers –2.00D, replace the +8.00D lens in the trial frame with a +6.00D lens.
- Now refined with +1.00D/–1.00D bracketing lenses.
- Eventually, fine tune with + 0.50D/–0.50D

Case Example: JND Cylinder Power and Axis

- Finding the best cylinder axis and power requires the same JND technique described above, now using a Jackson Cross Cylinder (JCC)
- For 20/50 or better vision, use a +/–0.25D JCC
- For 20/63 - 20/100, use a +/–0.50D JCC
- For 20/125 - 20/160, use a +/–0.75D JCC
- For 20/200 or less, use a +/–1.00D JCC

Case Example: JND Cylinder Power and Axis

- After establishing the spherical power as describe above, VA is 20/200
- 200/100 = 2.00D. Start with a +/–1.00 JCC
- With the JCC oriented for power at 90/180 degrees, ask the patient which is clearer.

- Patient states that +1.00D axis 180 is clearer. Put a +2.00D axis 180 cylinder lens in the trial frame.

- With a +2.00D axis 180 cylinder lens in the trial frame, again asked the patient to compare +1.00D to −1.00D axis 180. If the patient still prefers +1.00D axis 180, replace the +2.00D axis 180 cylinder lens in the trial frame with a +4.00D axis 180 cylinder lens.

- With a +4.00D axis 180 cylinder lens in the trial frame, again asked the patient to compare +1.00D to −1.00D axis 180. If the patient now prefers −1.00D axis 180, replace the +4.00D axis 180 cylinder lens in the trial frame with a +3.00D axis 180 cylinder lens.

- Now refined with a +0.50D/−0.50D JCC.

- Once the cylinder power is determined, repeat the same process to determine the cylinder axis.

Final Comments JND Refraction
- Remember to decreased power interval as visual acuity improves

- Use trial frame refraction when visual acuity is 20/50 or worse, or if regular refraction techniques are not working

- **The only intervention needed to enhance visual functioning may be to prescribe appropriate glasses**

An excellent refraction tutorial can be found online at
http://www.medrounds.org/refract/menu.htm
This tutorial will walk you though the various parts of a subjective refraction and will also provide you with a retinoscopy and refraction simulator.

41. **Contact Lenses**
by Ali Bukhamseen, OD, FAAO, FIACLE

Contact Lens Types

a. **Hard**: Any contact lens made of polymethylmethacralate (PMMA). This first contact lens style was invented in the 1940s. PMMA was an excellent material in terms of cost, chemical and physical stability, wetability and manufacturing ease. However, its inability to transmit oxygen ultimately limited its practical use.

b. **Gas Permeable (GP)**: Any contact lens made of a material that transmits a usable amount of oxygen and carbon dioxide. In the 1970s gas permeable contact lenses were developed. This lens style incorporated either silicon (siloxymethacrylates) or fluorine (fluorocarbon methacrylates) into the contact lens material. By doing this, oxygen was able to transmit through the lens material, making these lenses healthier for the eye than PMMA lenses. GP lenses were introduced into clinical practice in the 1980s after lens manufacturers had modified the ratios of methylmethacrylate, silicon, fluorine and various wetting agents to provide the best possible balance of oxygen permeability, wetability, dimensional stability and deposit resistance.

c. **Soft**: Any contact lens made of a water-absorbing substance which, when worn, is soft and flexible. In 1960s the first successful hydrogel material was developed (poly-2-hydroxyethyl methacrylate or polyHEMA). Hydrophilic polymeric materials are plasticized by the water they absorb. These materials have been used not only in contact lenses, but also in implant devices throughout the human body. Examples include foldable IOL, scleral buckle materials and drug delivery devices. The water content of these materials is around 38%. Methacrylic Acid (a negatively charged material) or Polyvinyl Alcohol (hydrophilic material) can be added to the hydrogel material to increase the water contents to 60% or more.

d. **Silicone Hydrogel**: This new generation of hydrogel contact lenses is made of silicone rubber combined with conventional hydrogel monomers. The silicone component provides extremely high oxygen permeability, while the hydrogel component facilitates fluid transport and lens movement.

There are four major lens wearing categories of hydrogel contact lenses:

- **Daily Wear**: This type of contact lenses is worn on a daily basis. These lenses are generally worn an average of 12 to 16 hours a day and removed before bedtime for cleaning and disinfection. These lenses are normally worn for 6 to 12 months before replacement.

- **Flexible Wear**: Flexible wear includes a variety of lens wearing schedules. Usually, this term indicates the patient wears their lenses overnight on an occasional basis.

- **Extended Wear**: This type of contact lens can be worn continuously for up to 30 days before they are replaced.

- **Planned Replacement**: There are five types of planned replacement, also called frequent replacement lenses; daily (used for one day only), weekly, bi-weekly, monthly, and quarterly replacement.

The primary difference between the aforementioned wearing categories is the lens's oxygen transmission capabilities.

Contact Lens Designs

a. **Spherical**: Any contact lens with an inside surface that is spherical.

b. **Toric**: Any contact lens with two different posterior surface curvatures.

c. **Bi-toric**: Any gas permeable contact lens where both surfaces (anterior and posterior) are toric. Usually fabricated so that the steepest radius of each surface lies in the same meridian.

d. **Bifocal**: Any contact lens having two different focal powers, one for distance vision and one for near vision.

e. **Bandage**: Any soft contact lenses used as a bandage on the cornea to protect it from air, foreign bodies, bacteria, or as a conveyor of medication.

f. **Cosmetic**: Any contact lens designed to alter or enhance the appearance of the eye (i.e. to conceal a disfigurement or to change its color). Cosmetic contact lenses may range from tinted lens to completely opaque lens with a painted pupil, iris, and sclera.

g.   **Bi-curve**: Any contact lens having two curvatures on its posterior surface.   The central, base curve forms the optic zone, and the other, a flatter curve forms the annular peripheral zone.

h.   **Fenestrated**: Any gas permeable contact lens containing one or more perforations for the more rapid transfer of air and/or tears between the contact lens and the cornea.

Properties of Contact Lens Materials

The most common physical and chemical properties for gas permeable and hydrogel contact lenses are:

a.   Oxygen Permeability/Transmission: Oxygen Permeability (Dk) is a property of the lens material that is independent of the size, shape, or surface condition of the lens.

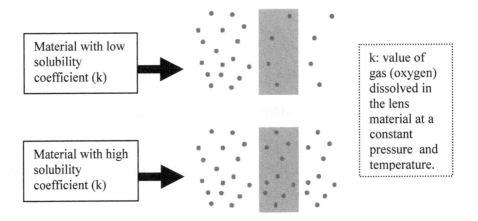

b.   Oxygen transmissibility (Dk/t) is a measure of the amount of oxygen transmitted through the lens. It is dependent on the Dk value of the material and the thickness (t) (typically center thickness) of the contact lens. With hydrogel contact lens materials, the Dk decreases logarithmically as the center thickness increases.

Example: If Dk value is 60 and the central thickness is 0.10 mm, the Dk/t is equal to 60. If the central thickness is 0.20 mm, the Dk/t decreases by a factor of 2 to a value of 30.

c. Another method of measuring oxygen transfer through GP lenses is Equivalent Oxygen Percentage (EOP). EOP is a measure of the amount of oxygen in the tears between the lens and the cornea and is determined in vivo. Essentially, it is a predictor of how much oxygen will reach the anterior corneal surface for a particular lens material and design. The maximum value is 21%.

d. Surface Wettability: Surface wettability is the ability of a blink to spread tear film mucin across the anterior contact lens surface. Wettability of a contact lens can be measured in several ways. The most famous one is the Sessile Drop test. In this test, a drop of pure water is placed on the test surface. The angle between the tangent to the drop's surface at the point of contact and the horizontal test surface is measured.

  i.   A zero angle: completely wettable
  ii.   A low angle: somewhat wettable
  iii. A large angle (> 90°): poorly wettable

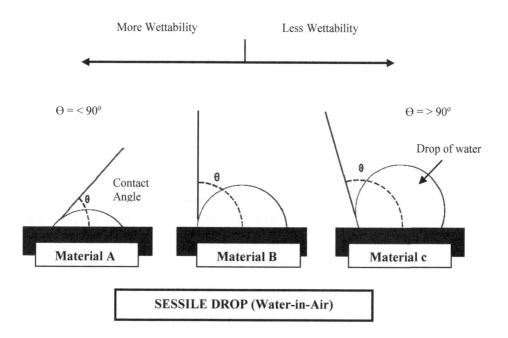

SESSILE DROP (Water-in-Air)

e.   Flexural Resistance: Flexural Resistance is the ability of GP lens to resist the bending or flexing forces on the lens when worn on a toric cornea. In other words, a lens with poor flexure resistance will tend to flex during the blinking process, inducing residual astigmatism.

f.   Water Content: Hydrogel contact lenses have water as their main content. The lens's properties of oxygen permeability, deposits resistance, flexibility and durability all depend on the water content of the lens. Oxygen permeability and flexibility increase as the water content increases, while deposits resistance and durability decrease. Most hydrogel lenses have water contents between 30% and 80% of their weight. Water content is classified as low (< 40%), medium (40% to 60%) and high (>60%).

Contact Lens Parameters

The main contact lens parameters are back optic zone radius, total diameter, back vertex power, and lens design (for gas permeable lenses).

a.   Back Optic Zone Radius (BOZR): Back optic zone radius or base curve is the curve of the posterior surface in the area corresponding to the optical zone.

b.   Total Diameter (TD): The liner measurement of the maximum external dimension of the contact lens. It is equal to the BOZR plus twice the width of each of the back peripheral optic zones (if any) or twice the width of the edge in a spherical lens.

c.   Back Vertex Power (BVP): The vergence power is expressed with reference to the posterior surface of the contact lens at the optical axis.

d.   Design: Describes the peripheral curve measurements and the finishing of GP lens edge. Peripheral curves encompass the outer 20% to 35% of a GP lens. The peripheral curve surrounds the optical zone diameter. The most common GP designs have either one (bicurve), two (tricurve), or three (tetracurve) peripheral curves. Some lens designs utilize an aspheric periphery to increase flexibility in dealing with a range of corneal contours.

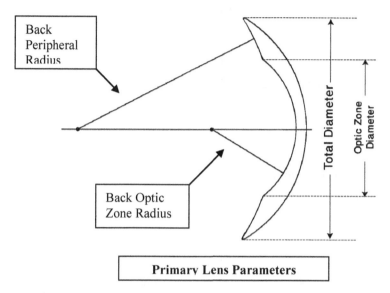

Primary Lens Parameters

Patient Assessment

a. Begins with the patient history. Contraindications for contact lens wear must be assessed with respect to general systemic conditions, systemic medications, allergies, previous ocular pathology and general ocular history. After the case history comes the refraction.

b. After the refractive error has been determined, the vertex distance must be corrected for when the refractive error is > +/- 4.00. Use the formula $F_{CL} = F_{spectacle}/(1-dF_{spectacle})$ (see page 153) to compensate for vertex distance.

   i. Example: What would the contact lens power be for a -6.50D sphere at a 12mm vertex distance?

$$F_{CL} = -6.50/(1- (0.012 \times -6.50)) = -6.50/(1 - (-0.078))$$
$$F_{CL} = -6.50/1.078 = -6.00 \text{ diopters}$$

   ii. It is important when dealing with astigmatic correction to treat both meridians independently by converting to cross cylinder form. Example: Refraction: -6.00-2.00x180 @ 12mm vertex distance

Cross cylinder:

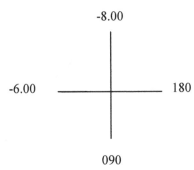

After vertex correction calculation:

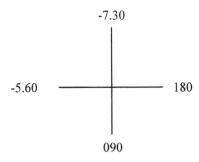

iii.   The minimum step in power of ophthalmic lenses or contact lenses is 0.25 diopter. Therefore, the powers will change to (-7.25 @ 90) and (-5.50@180).

iv.   Final toric contact lens power would be

-5.50 –1.75X180

c.   Anterior segment measurements: In fitting either gas permeable or soft contact lens, the following measurements should be recorded:

i.   Horizontal visible iris diameter (HVID): This measurement is used to ensure that a soft lens's total diameter is sufficient to maintain full cornea coverage.

ii.   Pupil size: This measurement allows the practitioner to predict, and manage, any likely flare from a misalignment of the pupil diameter with the back optic zone diameter of a GP lens. It is also important in fitting soft and GP bifocal contact lens.

    iii.   Tear prism height: The slit-lamp is used to judge the height of the inferior tear meniscus, which gives a useful guide to the volume of tears on the eye. A normal value would be 0.2 to 0.3 mm.

    iv.   Keratometry: It is important to record k-readings for all individuals being fit with contact lenses. K-readings have little correlation to soft contact lens fitting performance on normal corneas. However, it is the principle values used to select the initial trial lens for both soft and gas permeable contact lens. K-readings should be monitored on a regular basis. In addition to the values, the clarity of the mires should also be recorded. This gives an indication of corneal clarity and is a sensitive monitor of early corneal distortion.

    v.   Non-invasive break-up time (NIBUT)/ Tear thinning time (TTT): Keratometry can also be used to measure tear film stability. It is recorded as the time taken for the mire images to distort (TTT) and/or break up after a blink (NIBUT). Abnormal values are less than 10 seconds.

    vi.   Anterior segment exam: The slit lamp examination is the most important procedure in both pre-assessment and aftercare of contact lens wearer.

    vii.   Corneal topography: Allows the practitioners to measure the shape factor of the cornea. This can be used to help chose the lens design, including to what extent the peripheral curves of the lens need to flatten to maintain corneal alignment. Also, it is helpful to explain unusual fluorescein patterns or poorly centered lenses. Additionally, the principal meridians and degree of astigmatism can be shown at positions away from the central cornea, which is of value when fitting toric contact lenses.

Spherical Soft Contact Lens Fitting

The ideal soft contact lens fit should show the following characteristics:

    a.   Corneal coverage: The lens should cover the cornea in primary and secondary gaze at all times. Ideally, the contact lens should be larger than the HVID by 1 to 2 mm.

b. Dynamic fit: The lens must allow tear exchange to enable metabolic debris from the cornea to be removed. The amount of movement with each blink depends on the contact lens parameters as well as its thickness. Regular movement should be between 0.1 to 1.0 mm.

c. Alignment: The lens should align with the cornea and the conjunctiva and should show no indentation of conjunctival vessels that would indicate stagnation of tears in this area, potentially reducing oxygen supply to the limbus. Also, the lens should not show any edge stand off, which can lead to discomfort and excessive movement.

d. Centration: The lens should remain centered on the cornea in all position of gazes.

e. Patient feedback: When the above criteria are achieved, the patient should express comfort with crisp and clear vision.

Toric Soft Contact Lens Fitting

Toric contact lens can be fit empirically or with trial lenses. Torics are now available in thinner designs and higher water content, which improves the physiological performance of the lens on the eye. The key to successful soft toric fitting is the rotational stability of the lens. The interaction of the lids with the contact lens during the blink, induces rotation of the lens on the eye. To keep the astigmatic correction of the lens in alignment to that of the eye, the lens must be held in position. There are two basic ways to achieve this:

a. Prism stabilization: Is the most common means of stabilizing a contact lens. The lens is produced with a thicker edge profile towards its base. This causes the thinner portion of the lens to locate under the upper eyelid.

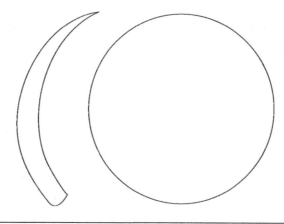

Cross-section through a prism-ballasted soft toric contact lens

b. Dynamic stabilization: Relies on the interaction between the lids and the lens to achieve stabilization. Stabilization is achieved by either designing thin zones superior and inferior to the optic zone or by placing two raised areas with orientation cams at the 3 and 9 o'clock position. The lids squeeze against the thickness differential, which creates rotational stability.

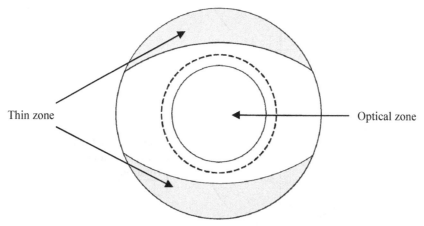

Thin zone   Optical zone

Dynamic Stabilizer design of soft toric contact lens

After a toric trial contact lens is inserted, the lens should be allowed to settle before the fit is assessed. Once settled, the practitioner looks for rotational stability. This is carried out by viewing the axis location marks on the lens. The practitioner notes the position of the rotation marks and judges the degree of rotation present (if any). This can be measured by rotating the slit beam on the slit lamp or by estimating the rotation by using the axis marks on the lenses as a guide. The axis rotation gives the information needed to order the next lens. The rotation shows how far the axis of the cylinder will need to be adjusted when ordering the final lens axis.

For example:

   i. Refraction: -4.00-2.25X180

  ii. Trial lens fitting: CL rotated clockwise by 10 degrees

 iii. Real correction: -4.00-2.25X170

 iv. Compensation: 10 degree counter clockwise

  v. Final axis: -4.00-2.25X010

 vi. 10 degrees clockwise rotation will bring the axis to 180 degree.

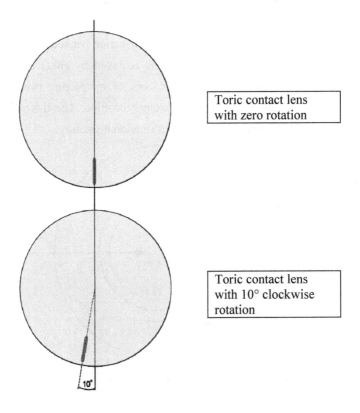

Toric contact lens with zero rotation

Toric contact lens with 10° clockwise rotation

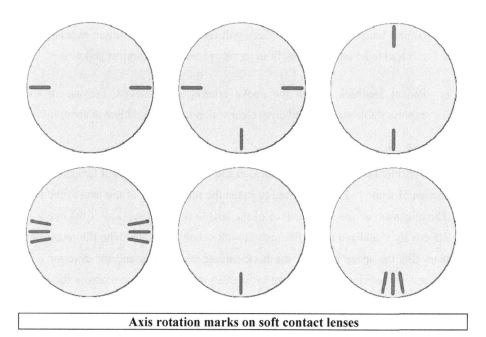

Axis rotation marks on soft contact lenses

Gas Permeable Contact Lens Fitting

As in soft contact lens fitting, the ideal GP fit should show the following characteristics:

a. Centration: The lens should remain centered over the pupil in primary gaze and maintain reasonable centration with each blink.

b. Corneal coverage: GP lens should in general be smaller than the corneal diameter. This smaller design will facilitate tear exchange under the lens and help optimize the alignment of the lens.

c. Dynamic fitting: GP lens should move to enable oxygen exchange via the tear pump. Lens movement is one of the key characteristics of an ideal GP fit. The lens should move 1 to 1.5 mm with each blink. Excessive movement causes patient discomfort, inconsistent vision and may be associated with conjunctival staining.

d. Alignment: The ideal GP fit should show alignment of the back surface of the lens with the cornea over most of the lens surface. A narrow band of edge clearance at the lens periphery is required to enable adequate tear exchange and to facilitate lens removal. The alignment of the back surface with the cornea allows the force of the lens to be distributed across the maximum bearing surface of the cornea. However, slight apical clearance and an area of light corneal touch in the mid-periphery will enhance lens centration: excessive touch can lead to an unstable lens fit in terms of centration, comfort and vision.

e. Patient feedback: When the above criteria are achieved, the patient should express stable comfort and crisp clear vision following patient adaptation.

Slit Lamp Evaluation of GP Lenses

The dynamic fit of GP lenses is assessed and measured using a slit lamp. An optical section of white light can be used to judge the relationship of the lens to the cornea. The alignment of the back surface of the lens to the front surface of the eye is most effectively visualized using fluorescein with cobalt blue light. The fluorescein in the tears fills the space between the back surface of the lens and the anterior corneal surface. By looking at the change in intensity of the fluorescein across the lens, the distance between the posterior lens surface and the anterior corneal surface can be visualized. This is called the fluorescein pattern.

Tear Lens

The tear lens is formed by the tear film between the posterior surface of the contact lens and the anterior surface of the cornea. If the tear film has a uniform thickness, as with a soft contact lens, it has a Plano power. For GP lenses, fitting with a steeper base curve produces a tear lens that will be thicker in the middle, creating a positive powered tear lens. The opposite occurs when fitting with a flatter base curve, which creates a negative powered tear lens. Additionally, tear lens allows a spherical GP lens to neutralize corneal astigmatism.

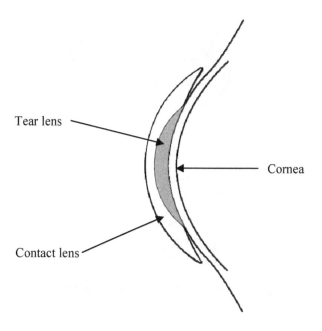

Presbyopia

There are many types of bifocal contact lenses on the market. The following are the bifocal designs available today:

a. Alternating bifocal: The alternating or translating bifocal was one of the first types of bifocal contact lens to be produced. The patient looks through the distance portion of the optic zone in primary gaze. On down gaze, the lens is held up against the lower eyelid, to allow for viewing through the near portion of the lens.

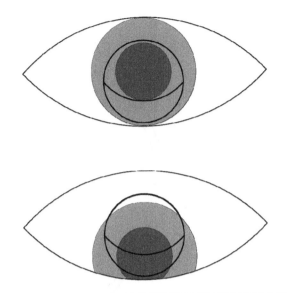

The principle of the translating bifocal contact lens

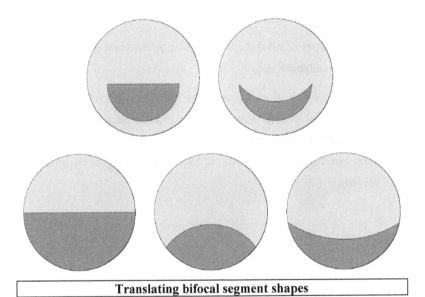

Translating bifocal segment shapes

b. Simultaneous vision designs: simultaneous bifocal designs rely on an optical system that place two images on the retina simultaneously. The visual system then selects the clearer image. The power distribution across the lens surface is variable and these lenses have been described as multifocal, aspheric or progressive. This lens design is available in soft and GP material.

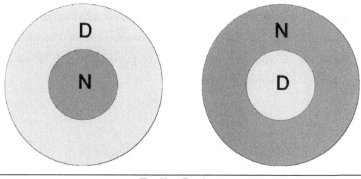

Earlier Designs
Bi-centric center-near design (left)
Bi-centric center-distance design (right)

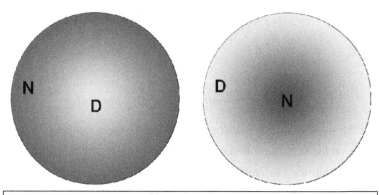

Newer Designs
Back surface center-distance design (left)
Front surface center-near design (right)

c. Aspheric center-distance: These lenses have a back aspheric curve with the central portion of the lens's optical zone focused for distance vision, while the surrounding area contains the power required for near work. Rays of light from a distant object are focusing by the central zone. When the object is at near, the reverse occurs. The light rays from the peripheral zone are now in focus on the retina. The visual system attends to the clearer of the two images.

d. Aspheric center-near: The center-near focused aspheric bifocal was introduced to address the problem of pupil constriction during near viewing. The optical principle is the same as for the center-distance focused lens, only in reverse. With this lens, the central portion of the lens focuses the image from close objects while the surrounding area is used for distance viewing.

e. Multi-zone concentric (center and distance): This lens design consisting of five alternating concentric distance and near powered zones. The width and spacing of the zones is based on the variation of pupil size in different illuminations within the presbyopic population.

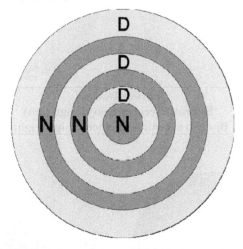

Multi-zone concentric center distance design

f. Diffractive bifocal: diffractive lenses work on the principle of placing a phase plate on the surface of the lens. The phase plate is able to split the light passing through into two discrete focal points, one for distance and the other for near. With this design, the performance of the lens becomes independent of pupil size as long as the pupil diameter remains smaller than the diffractive zone in the lens.

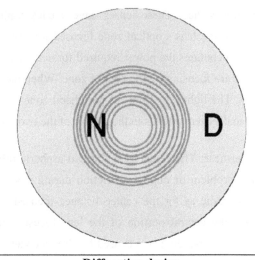

Diffractive design

Aphakia

The quality of vision with contact lens is typically very good for aphakes. In comparison, spectacles tend to create visual distortions that can be upsetting to the wearers. Most aphakes will sacrifice a line or two of Snellen acuity in exchange for the better field of vision that contact lens provides. Astigmatism often occurs in aphakic eyes due to surgery. The simplest solution is to correct this with GP lenses. But, if the patient can not tolerate a PG lens, a soft lens may be used. If an astigmatic correction is needed, it can be provided in spectacles worn over the contact lenses. Because the aphake requires a near addition, bifocal spectacles can be used to correct the astigmatism at the same time.

Keratoconus

The progression of keratoconus varies with each individual. Once the individual no longer has clear vision with spectacles, they will be fit with GP lenses. Limitations of spectacle corrections with keratoconus include irregular corneal astigmatism and frequent changes of refractive error.

a.   GP lenses are the lens of choice for keratoconus. The GP lens creates a spherical, regular refracting surface that results in improved visual acuity.

b.   Fitting keratoconus with GP lenses depends on: type of cone, amount of steepening, lid characteristics, quantity and quality of tears, and patient adaptation.

c.   There are three types of cones described in keratoconus: the nipple cone (smaller than 5 mm), the oval cone, and the globus cone (greater than 6 mm).

   i.   The nipple cone is steep, round, and located in the inferior nasal paracentral area of the cornea.

   ii.   The oval cone is similar to the nipple cone, but it is slightly larger and more oval, and the apex decenters inferiotemporally.

   iii.   The globus cone is the largest cone and is more diffuse.

d.   The most common lens designs used in keratoconus fitting are the three-point touch, apical clearance, the piggyback system and aspheric lens.

i. Three-point touch design

Three-point touch design describes a GP lens that is fit with three areas of light touch. These areas are located at the apex and two other points in the midperiphery. This type of design distributes the support of the lens over a large area of the cornea.

ii. Apical clearance design

This lens design vaults the central cornea and bears on the corneal periphery. It is assumed that a lens that vaults the cornea will not produce central scarring.

iii. Piggyback system

This design describes the technique of fitting a GP lens on top of a soft lens. This method is used to increase patient comfort, enhance lens centration, and add protection to the apex of the cone. Because corneal sensitivity increases with keratoconus, some patient will reject a GP lens even when it improves their visual acuity. Wearing a soft contact lens under a GP lens will increase patient comfort. To avoid corneal hypoxia, ultra thin, high water content soft contact lens must be used. Also, the GP lens should be made of a high oxygen permeable material.

iv. Aspheric design

Aspheric lenses become progressively flatter from the center to the periphery. This provides better alignment on the cornea, which is also aspheric in shape. Ideally the lens should touch the cone with complete peripheral clearance and minimal movement with the blink.

Post-Operative Keratoplasty

Soft contact lens may be used to aid in wound healing; however, adequate visual acuity is usually not obtained with soft lenses when significant irregular astigmatism is present. The lens of choice is a high Dk GP lens. In some cases a bitoric GP lens may be necessary to correct high amount of astigmatism. The contact lens will need to be large enough to cover the host-graft junction and provide minimal bearing on this area.

Contact Lens References:

1. Jones L. Modern Contact Lens Materials: A Clinical Performance Update, *Contact Lens Spectrum* 2002;17(9):24-35;

2. International Association of Contact Lens Educators. Module 2: Introduction to Contact Lenses, Module 3: Contact Lens Fitting, and Module 6: The Cornea in Contact Lens. *IACLE Contact Lens Course.* Sydney, NSW, Australia: International Association of Contact Lens Educators, 2006.

3. Veys J, Meyler J, Davies I. *Essential Contact Lens Practice.* Oxford, Boston: Butterworth-Heinemann, 2002.

4. Bennett E. Weissman E, eds. *Clinical Contact Lens Practice.* Philadelphia: Lippincott Williams & Wilkins, 2005.

42.   Vision Rehabilitation

Introduction

Vision rehabilitation encompasses the management of individuals of all ages, who have a congenital or acquired impairment of visual acuity and/or visual field and/or other functionally disabling factors, in the better seeing eye, in which the loss of vision interferes with the process of learning, vocational or avocational pursuits, social interaction, or the activities of daily living. This vision loss cannot be adequately improved by conventional refractive measures.

Vision rehabilitation involves a continuum of care, which begins with medical and surgical intervention and proceeding through to the prescription of low vision devices and vision rehabilitation services. Vision rehabilitation is an intervention intended to maximize the use of residual vision and provide the individual with practical adaptations for their normal activities of daily living and any other desired tasks. As the result of the vision rehabilitation process, the individual will attain the maximum function of their remaining vision, a sense of well-being and a personally satisfying level of independence.

Maximum functioning is achieved through the use of optical, non-optical, and/or video magnification devices or by teaching of compensatory non-visual techniques. Vision rehabilitation may be necessitated by any condition, disease or injury that causes a visual impairment serious enough to result in functional limitations or disability. There is no required amount of visual acuity or visual field loss necessary, before an individual can be referred for low vision rehabilitation. The process of vision rehabilitation is felt to be more effective if it is started as soon as functional visual difficulties are identified. This will allow the low vision rehabilitation team the opportunity to minimize the resultant visual disability and subsequent visual handicap. The vision rehabilitation team may include, but is not limited to, medical, optometric, allied health, social, educational and psychological services.

Definitions

    a. "Visual Function" measures how the eye and visual system function, as determined by visual acuity and visual field measurements.

    b. "Functional Vision" refers to how the person functions with everyday activities. Functional vision takes into account factors such as loss of contrast sensitivity, photophobia, and/or ocular motor problems.

(Source: American Medical Association's Guidelines Evaluation of Permanent Impairment, 5th Edition, 2001)

c.   Functional definition of low vision/visual impairment:

"Low Vision" is a visual impairment, not correctable by standard glasses, contact lenses, medicine, or surgery, that interferes with the person's ability to perform every day activities.

(Source: www.nei.nih.gov/nehep/nehepov.htm)

d.   Legally Blind (United States)

"Remaining vision in the better eye after best correction is less than 20/100 OR contraction of the peripheral visual fields in the better eye (A) to 10 degrees or less from the point of fixation; or (B) so the widest diameter subtends an angle no greater than 20 degrees."

(Source: www.ssa.gov/disability/professionals/bluebook/2.00-SpecialSensesandSpeech-adult.htm)

The World Health Organization defines legal blindness as visual acuity less than 20/400 and/or a field of vision of 10 degrees or less.

Magnification/Reading Add Estimation Techniques

Determining Needed Magnification

Magnification needs are based on the initial reference value and the desired final value. Clinically, it is the entrance distance or near acuity divided by the goal acuity (VA/VA').

Magnification Estimation Techniques (Reading add/reading spectacles)

Accurate near visual acuity testing is essential in determining magnification needs for reading and other near point activities.

Kestenbaum's Rule: To determine the power necessary to read 1M print (newsprint), take the reciprocal of the distance acuity to establish a starting add power.

Example   20/50 — 50/20 = +2.50D Add
                       20/200 — 200/20 = +10.00D Add
                       20/400 — 400/20 = +20.00D Add

Because distance acuity is a poor predictor of near visual functioning, this is the least accurate method of determining reading add power.

Lighthouse Add Determination: To determine the power needed to read 1M print, measure the patients near acuity at a 16 inch/40 cm working distance (WD). Multiply the M acuity by 2.50D to arrive at the theoretical add power needed to read 1M print

> Example   4M @ 40cm/16 inches — 2.50 x 4 = 10.00D Add
>
>   2M @ 40cm/16 inches — 2.50 x 2 = 5.00D Add

The Lighthouse method establishes the starting power. An individual may need additional power if their contrast sensitivity is reduced, they have multiple scotomas, they need to read print smaller than 1M or they have less than ideal illumination when reading. The clinician should adjust the add power using normal reading materials under task lighting to determine how much add is actually needed.

Optical Devices

To prescribe the appropriate low vision devices, it critical to determine the magnification required and understand the optical properties of the systems being considered. The optical properties include the depth of field (object plane), weight, cost and cosmesis of the various devices being considered.

Sequence of Device Presentation

- Spectacles
- Hand/Stand Magnifiers
- Telescopes (hand held and spectacle mounted)
- Absorptive Lenses
- Electronic
- Non-Optical

Regular Spectacles as determined by a trial frame refraction.
- For distance acuity improvement
- For near/intermediate tasks, where lower magnification is required
- To use with optical devices. It is important to remember that stand magnifiers require accommodation or add, and have maximum add limitations
- CCTVs may require accommodation or add for the working distance

Stronger bifocal corrections will be required to use relative distance magnification early in the vision loss process. As higher amounts of reading addition are needed (>6D), a +4.00D add may prove beneficial as an intermediate distance add for these individuals. Individuals benefiting from this type of intermediate correction are those that need lower amounts of magnification for less detailed tasks such as signing their name, cutting their finger nails, seeing the food on their plate as well as cooking and reading larger print, such as the headlines, etc.

Spectacle Magnifiers
- Prismatic half eye readers (+4.00 to +12.00D with base in prism)
- High plus aspheric readers (+10.00 to +20.00D)
- Microscopic spectacles (2x (8D) to 12x (48D) in aspheric or doublet design)
- Specialty microscopic spectacles, in powers to 80D, are available in doublet lens systems, wide-angle microscopic lenses and high-add bifocals.
- Press on adds are available as 22mm bifocal segments in powers from 8 to 40D
- Clip-on and head borne loupes are also available in various powers

When prescribing reading spectacles, is important to consider whether the patient functions better monocularly or binocularly. If patient is monocular they will not need prism incorporated into their reading spectacles and they may need to occlude/fog their fellow eye if it interferes with the better eye. For those individuals who have similar near acuities between their two eyes and whose binocular acuity is better or the same as their monocular acuity, base in prism will provide more comfortable, sustained reading abilities. Base in prism is used for adds of +4.00 to +12.00D. The prism power equals the add strength + 2 prism diopters Base In, in each eye. For example a +6.00D add would have 8 prism diopters Base In, added to each eye.

Advantages-Spectacle Magnifiers
- Frees the hands for manipulative tasks
- Provides widest field of vision of equivalent powered optical options
- Allows greater reading speed of equivalent powered reading options (once adapted)
- Makes binocular vision possible to approximately a 10.00 diopter add equivalent
- More cosmetically acceptability to some individuals than other options
- Portable and relatively inexpensive

Disadvantages-Spectacle Magnifiers
- Requires closer working distance and may obstruct illumination
- May be inconvenient for spot reading task, where information is gained from single words or short phrases (e.g. price tags)
- Fixed optical center may reduce effectiveness when using eccentric fixation
- Makes writing difficult if lens add is stronger than 10.00 diopters
- Working distance as determined by taking the reciprocal of the equivalent add power (+20D lens will have the working distance of 100/20 = 5cm)

Magnifiers

Hand Magnifiers
- Hand magnifiers are positioned so that the materials being viewed are at the focal point of the lens.
- Hand magnifiers are used with the individual's distance spectacle correction.
- Hand magnifiers come in both illuminated (standard bulbs or LED bulbs) or non illuminated versions.
- Patients need to be made aware that the larger the lens diameter, the weaker the lens power.

Hand magnifier considerations include the optical design; spherical, aspheric/Bi-aspheric which are thinner, lighter, flatter; or aplanatic doublet. Other considerations include illumination source and ergonomics.

Conventional lenses have a front surface that is spherical. Aspheric lenses have a complex front surface that gradually changes curve from the center of the lens to the edge. For aspheric hand magnifiers, the front surface gradually flattens toward the edge of the lens. Aspheric lens designs reduce or eliminate distortions induced when looking away from the optical center of the lens. Aspheric designed lenses have directionality. This means that the more curved surface should face toward the individual using it.

Aplanatic magnifier systems are created by two plano-convex lenses whose convex surfaces face each other. This results in a distortion free image up to the edge of the lens.

Advantages-Hand Magnifiers
- User can read at a more customary/longer working distance than comparable powered reading spectacles

- Large range of magnification available
- Low patient resistance (familiar device/cosmetically acceptable)
- Convenient for spot reading task, when information is gained from single words or short phrases (e.g. price tags)
- Available with built in light source to enhance contrast
- Generally inexpensive, portable, and usable with the individual's spectacle correction

Disadvantages-Hand Magnifiers
- Must be held with one hand (sometimes 2)
- Prolonged reading can be slow and uncomfortable
- Extended use causes hand and arm fatigue and reduced field of view slows reading
- Must be held at correct focal distance to obtain maximum power
- Less effective for individuals with limited dexterity or hand tremors
- Illuminated versions require batteries

Stand Magnifiers
- Available in illuminated and non illuminated designs
- The larger the lens diameter, the weaker the lens power
- Stand magnifiers need to be used with a reading correction

Advantages-Stand Magnifiers
- Available in very strong powers (88D)
- Eye to lens distance can be varied
- Magnification is constant for a given add power
- Suitable with limited dexterity/hand tremors
- Useable at normal reading distances
- Useful for individuals with constricted visual fields when held at arm's length
- Available with built in light source to enhance contrast
- Useable with standard reading adds
- Generally light weight, portable and inexpensive

Disadvantages-Stand Magnifier
- Less convenient to carry due to size
- Requires one or both hands
- More bulky than hand magnifiers
- Awkward to use on non-flat surfaces

- Field of vision is smaller than equivalent powered spectacle lenses
- Causes excessive shading and reduces lighting onto surface (unless self-illuminated)
- Impossible to write under most designs
- Prolonged use may result in poor posture
- The individual's bifocal strength may not match the image plane of the stand magnifier
- Illuminated versions require batteries or direct current

Telemicroscopes (a.k.a. reading telescopes or surgical loupes)
- Can be hand-held or spectacle mounted
- Spectacle mounted in a full diameter (center mounting) or bioptic configuration
- Available in Galilean or Keplerian design

Advantages-Telemicroscopes
- Useful for a wide range of focusing distances, from far to near
- Allows greater working distance than equivalent powered microscopic spectacles
- Spectacle mounted design affords hands free magnification
- Auto focus versions available
- Binocularity possible for fixed focusing distance

Disadvantage-Telemicroscopess
- Smaller field of view than equivalent powered microscopic spectacles
- Reduces image brightness through the telescope
- Depth of focus more critical, requiring stability of working distance
- Weight
- Cosmesis
- Relatively expensive

Telescopes
- Hand held or spectacle mounted
- Monocular or binocular
- Galilean or Keplerian
- Fixed focus, manual focus and auto focus systems are available
- For distance, intermediate or near vision enhancement

Telescopes are afocal optical systems consisting of two lenses, separated in space. The lenses are separated by the sum of their focal lengths.

Galilean telescopes have a (+) objective lens and a (-) ocular lens. Galilean telescopes form an erect/upright image.

Keplerian telescopes have a (+) object of lens and a (+) ocular lens. Keplerian (astronomical) telescopes form an inverted image so they require an erecting lens or prisms to make it a terrestrial telescope.

Galilean telescopes have several practical advantages for vision rehabilitation work. The image is upright, without the need for image erecting prisms and the device is shorter. Galilean telescopes typically are 2, 3 or 4x in strength, inexpensive, light, and have a large exit pupil, which makes centering less difficult.

4x telescopes and stronger are usually Keplerian in design which gives an optically superior image, but are more expensive with a smaller exit pupil requiring better centering and aiming. Keplerian binoculars, contain prisms to erect the otherwise inverted image.

Galilean telescopes used as surgical loupes, require an add to be combined with the objective lens. The field size is far smaller than that obtained with bifocal spectacles.

Advantages-Telescopes
- Useful for magnification from near to distance
- Useful for specific tasks requiring magnification at variable distances
- Portable monocular units are useful for spot distance vision (e.g. signs)
- Can be mounted in a spectacle to leave hands free if necessary

Disadvantages-Telescopes
- Field of view is restricted.
- The higher the power of the telescope, the smaller the field of view.
- Luminance is reduced because there is a 4% loss of light to reflection at every lens surface. This is reduced to some degree with the use of antireflective coatings.
- Depth of field is more narrowed compared to spectacle or hand held magnifiers for near use.
- Contrast is reduced when looking through a telescope. This can be a problem for individuals who have experienced a reduction in their contrast sensitivity.
- Often relatively expensive (spectacle mounted)

Video Magnification Devices

Closed Circuit TV (CCTV)

Advantages-CCTV

- Provides maximum contrast enhancement
- Allows binocularity at high levels of magnification
- Allows writing to be performed
- Provides wider field of view for level of magnification then standard magnifiers
- Allows sufficient reading speed to make continuous text meaningful at high levels of magnification
- Level of magnification can be easily adjusted for different sizes of materials or fluctuations in vision
- Suitable for individuals with physical impairments, loss of dexterity or hand tremors

Disadvantages-CCTV

- Less portable than other devices (although portable devices are now available)
- More expensive than other devices
- Some orientation and training may be required

Head Borne Video Magnification Devices

Advantages- Head Borne Video Magnification Devices
- Provides variable levels of magnification for near, intermediate and distance tasks
- Provides contrast enhancement
- Allows binocularity at high levels of magnification
- Allows manipulative tasks to be performed with both hands
- Level of magnification can be easily adjusted for different sizes of materials or fluctuations in vision
- Can provide direct input from the television

Disadvantages- Head Borne Video Magnification Devices
- Somewhat heavy when worn for extended periods of time
- Requires relatively good head control (no senescent tremors)
- More expensive than other devices
- Some orientation and training may be required

Absorptive Lenses

Advantages – Absorptive lenses
- Blocks UV
- Reduces glare
- Improves contrast
- May improve acuity

Disadvantages – Absorptive lenses
- May reduce acuity
- Alters color values

Glare Control
- Environmental Modifications
- Absorptive Filters
- Reflective Coatings
- Interference Coatings
- Special Lighting
- Visors/Caps
- Masking Devices

Non-Optical Devices
- Enlarged playing cards
- Enlarged bingo cards
- Bold rule paper
- Bold tipped pens
- Talking clocks/watches/calculator
- Enlarged faced thermostat dials
- Reading stands
- Level indicators
- Task lighting
- Large print reading materials
- Large print devices
- Telephones with large print buttons/displays
- Writing templates
- Signature guides
- Reading stands/clipboards

- o   Helpful for maintaining proper placement of reading materials when critical
- o   Reduces postural fatigue
- o   Facilitates adequate light on reading materials
- Typoscopes
  - o   Reduces glare from glossy paper
  - o   Minimizes figure ground confusion

Some make use of relative size magnification which can be used in conjunction with other forms of magnification (i.e. use of low powered reading lenses with large print)

There are a variety of options available, especially for ADLs

Illumination

Is the single most important factor in enhancing visual functioning.   The median illumination found to give optimum performance in a low vision clinic was 1188 lux, while the normal home conditions have a median value of only 177 lux.   More than 90% of low vision patients showed some improvement in near or distance visual acuity when the illumination was improved.   (Silver JH, Gould ES, Irvine D, Cullinan TR, Visual Acuity at Home and in Eye Clinics, Trans. Ophthalmol. Soc. UK (1978) 98: 262-266)

Types of illumination
- Incandescent
- Fluorescent
- Halogen

Light fixtures
- Are as important as the bulb
- Must be flexible to allow proximity to paper and a non-glaring angle
- Adjust position of light source for maximum comfort/contrast enhancement

Adaptive Technology

A comprehensive review of adaptive technology is beyond the scope of this presentation. What follows is a brief review of computer accessibility. Computer accessibility includes the following:

a.   Screen Enlarging Software

   b.   Screen Reading Software

   c.   Operating System Software

   d.   Text to Speech Software

Vision Rehabilitation References

   a.   Vision Problems in the US-2002, Prevalence of Adult Vision Impairment and Age Related Eye Disease, Demographics of Visual Impairment, 4th edition, National Eye Institute, Prevent Blindness America.
        (Source: www.usvisionproblems.org)

   b.   The Lighthouse Ophthalmology Resident Training Manual – A New Look at Low Vision Care, Faye, Albert, Freed, Seidman, Fischer (2000) Lighthouse International

   c.   Low Vision Rehabilitation: Caring for the Whole Person – Ophthalmology Monographs - 12, (1999), American Academy of Ophthalmology.

   d.   American Academy of Ophthalmology Preferred Practice Pattern, Rehabilitation: The Management of Adult Patients with Low Vision (1998), American Academy of Ophthalmology.

   e.   Optics, Refraction, and Contacts Lenses, Basic and Clinical Science Course, Section 3 (2004-2005), American Academy of Ophthalmology.

   f.   Foundations of Low Vision, Clinical and Functional Perspectives, Corn & Koenig, (1996) AFB Press.

   g.   Foundations of Rehabilitation Counseling with Persons who are Blind or Visually Impaired, Moore, Graves & Patterson, (1997) AFB Press.

   h.   Foundations of Orientation and Mobility, Second Edition, Blasch, Wiener & Welsh, (1997) AFB Press.

   i.   Visual Impairments: Determining Eligibility for Social Security Benefits (2002) Board on Behavioral, Cognitive, and Sensory Sciences and Education, National Research Council, National Academies Press.
        (Source: http://www.nap.edu/books/0309083486/html/)

   j.   Clinical Low Vision, Second Edition, Faye, (1984) Little, Brown & Company.

   k.   Vision and Aging, General and Clinical Perspectives, Second Edition, Rosenbloom and Morgan, (1993) Butterworth-Heinemann.

l. The Lighthouse Handbook on Vision Impairment in Vision Rehabilitation, Silverstone, Lang, Rosenthal, Faye, (2000) Oxford University Press.

m. Remediation and Management of Low Vision, Cole and Rosenthal, (1996) Mosby.

n. The Art and Practice of Low Vision, Second Edition, Freeman and Jose, (1997) Butterworth-Heinemann.

43.   Formulas at a Glance

Simple Lens Formula

U + D = V or 100/u (cm) + D = 100/v (cm)

Where: U = vergence of object at the lens   u = object   position

= 100/U (cm)

D = lens power

V = vergence of image rays   v = image   position

= 100/V (cm)

Lens Effectivity

The change in vergence of light that occurs at different points along its path. This is related to vertex distance.

Formula: $F_{new} = F_{current}/(1-dF_{current})$

Where F is in Diopters and d is in meters.

Optical Media and Indices of Refraction

Object vergence V = n/u

Image vergence V' =n'/u'

Where: n = index of refraction for where the light is coming from

n' = index of refraction for where the light is going to

u = object distance

u' = image distance

Snell's Law of Refraction

n sin i = n' sin r

Where: i = angle of incidence as measured from the normal

r = angle refracted as measured from the normal

n = index of refraction for where the light is coming from

n' = index of refraction for where the light is going to

Critical Angle

$\sin i_c = n'/n \times 1$

Where: i_c = the critical angle and the refracted angle is $90°$

  n = index of refraction for where the light is coming from

  n' = index of refraction for where the light is going to

Apparent Thickness Formula

$n/u = n'/u'$

Where: n = index of refraction for where the light is coming from

  n' = index of refraction for where the light is going to

  u = object distance

  u' = image distance

Mirrors

The focal length of a curved mirror is always ½ its radius of curvature ($f = r/2$)

The reflecting power of a mirror in diopters $D_M = 1/f\,(m)$

For mirrors or reflecting surfaces: $U + 2/r_m = V$, (r_m is in meters) or $U + 1/f = V$

Where: f = focal length of the mirror in meters

  r = radius of curvature of the mirror in meters

Prism Diopters

A Prism Diopter ($^\Delta$) is defined as a deviation of 1 cm at 1 meter.

Approximation Formula

For angles under $45°$ (or 100^Δ), each degree ($°$) of angular deviation equals approximately 2^Δ

Prentice's Rule

Deviation in prism diopters (PD) = h (cm) x F

Where: F = power of the lens

h = distance from the optical center of the lens

Convergence

Convergence $(^\Delta)$ = 100/working distance (cm) x Pupillary Distance (cm)

Convergence (in prism diopters) required for an ametrope to bi-fixate a near object is equal to the dioptric distance from the object to the center of rotation of the eyes, multiplied by the subject's intra-pupillary distance in centimeters.

Spherical Equivalent

Spherical equivalent = ½ cylinder power + sphere power

Relative Distance Magnification

Relative Distance Magnification = r/d

Where: r = reference or original working distance

d = new working distance

Relative Size Magnification

Relative Size Magnification = S2/S1

Where: S1 = original size

S2 = the new size

Transverse/Linear Magnification

$M_T = I/O = U/V = v/u$

Where: I = Image size

       O = Object size

       U = Object vergence

       V = Image vergence

       u = object distance

       v = image distance

Axial Magnification

$M_A = M_1 \times M_2$

$M_A = (M)^2$ (Approximation formula for Axial Magnification of objects with relatively small axial dimensions)

Rated Magnification

$M_r = F/4$

Assumes that the individual can accommodate up to 4.00 diopters when doing close work which gives d = 25cm (25cm is the standard reference distance used when talking about magnification).

Effective Magnification

$M_e = dF$

Where: d = reference distance in meters to the object (image is formed at infinity)

      F = the lens power

Conventional Magnification

$M_c = dF + 1$

Where: d = reference distance in meters to the object (image is formed at infinity)

F = the lens power

The underlying assumption in this equation is that the patient is "supplying" one unit (1X) of magnification

Angular Magnification of a Telescope

$M_{A \text{ Telescope}} = (-) F_E/F_O$

Where: F_E = eyepiece lens power

F_O = objective lens power

Accommodation through a Telescope Formula

(for accommodation required to view a near object through an afocal telescope)

$A_{oc} = M^2 U$

Where: A_{oc} = vergence at the eyepiece = accommodation
U = object vergence at the objective = 1/u
M = the magnification of the telescope

Aniseikonia

Total Magnification of a Lens: $M_{T} = M_P + M_S$.

Where: M_P is the magnification from the lens power
M_S is the magnification from the lens shape

Magnification from Power (M_P): $M_P = D_V H$

Where: D_V is the dioptric power of the lens
H is the vertex distance measured in cm

Magnification from Shape (M_S): $M_S = D_1 (t_{cm}/1.5)$

Where: D_1 is the curvature of the front surface of the lens

        t = the center thickness of the lens

        The 1.5 in the following equation is the index of refraction (approximately) of glass or plastic

IOL Power (SRK Formula)

$D_{IOL} = A - 2.5L - 0.9K$

Where: D_{IOL} = recommended power for emmetropia

        A = a constant (provided by manufacturers for their lenses)

        L = axial length in mm

        K = average keratometry reading in diopters for desired ametropia

Lens Clock

To calculate true power of a single refracting surface (SRS) using a lens clock

$F_{true} = F_{lens\ clock} (n'_{true} - n)/(n'_{lens\ clock} - n)$

Where: n'_{true} = the true index of refraction of the lens being measured

        $n'_{lens\ clock}$ = 1.53 (crown glass)

        n = 1.00 (air)

Ophthalmoscopic Magnification

Direct: $M = F/4$

Where: F = the total refractive power of the eye. The image is upright.

Indirect: $M_A = (-)D_{Eye}/C_{ondensing\ lens}$

The image of the fundus becomes the object of the condensing lens, which then forms an aerial image that is larger and inverted.

Astigmatism Estimation from Keratometry

Take the amount of with the rule astigmatism noted by keratometry readings, multiply that by 1.25, and then subtract that number from 0.75 diopters (lenticular astigmatism) to arrive at the estimated amount of refractive astigmatism.

When against the rule astigmatism is noted by keratometry, add 0.75 diopters to the full amount of corneal astigmatism to arrive at the estimated amount of refractive astigmatism.

Reflecting Power of the cornea to determine corneal curvature

$D = (n{-}1)/r$

Where: D is the reflecting power of the cornea
              n is the standardize refractive index of the cornea (1.3375)

Lens Tilt

The change in power of the sphere through tilting is determined by the formula:

$F (1 + 1/3 \sin^2 a)$

The created cylinder power is determined by the formula: $F (\tan^2 a)$

Where: a = the angle of tilt

A simplified formula to determine the change in sphere power is to take (1/10 the amount of tilt)^2 = the percentage of power added to the original sphere.

The increase in the cylindrical correct is approximately equal to 3x the induced sphere increase.

44. Optics Review Problem Set

Subject: Vergence – Formula U = 100/u where u is in centimeters

1) Light is traveling from right to left in air. Light converges 10 cm to right of a reference point. What is the vergence?
    a. +5.00D
    b. +10.00D
    c. −5.00D
    d. −10.00D
    e. −1.00D

2) Light is traveling from left to right in air. Light diverges from a point 20 cm to right of a reference point. What is the vergence?
    a. +5.00D
    b. +10.00D
    c. −5.00D
    d. −10.00D
    e. +1.00D

3) A pencil of rays converges toward a point 50 cm to the right of a lens. What is the vergence of light rays 15 cm to the right of the lens?
    a. +2.00D
    b. −2.00D
    c. +2.86D
    d. +6.67D
    e. −6.67D

4) A pencil of rays converges toward a point 50 cm to the right of a lens. What is the vergence of light rays 40 cm to the right of the lens?
    a. +2.50D
    b. +2.00D
    c. −10.00D
    d. +10.00D
    e. −2.50D

5) A pencil of rays converges toward a point 50 cm to the right of a lens. What is the vergence of light rays 55 cm to the right of the lens?

    a. −1.82D
    b. +1.82D
    c. +20.00D
    d. −20.00D
    e. +2.00D

6) Pencils of rays converge toward a point 50-cm to the right of a lens. What is the vergence of light rays 150 cm to the right of the lens?

    a. +2.00D
    b. −1.00D
    c. +1.00D
    d. −2.00D
    e. −2.50D

Subject: Effectivity - Formula: $F(new) = F(current)/(1-dF(current))$ where F is in diopters and d is in meters

7) A pencil of rays emerges from a lens with a vergence of +6 D. What is the vergence after a travel of 10 mm in air?

    a. +15.00D
    b. +6.38D
    c. +5.66D
    d. −6.38D
    e. −5.66D

8) A pencil of rays emerges from a lens with a vergence of −8 D. What is the vergence after a travel of 15 mm in air?

    a. +7.14D
    b. −7.14D
    c. −3.63D
    d. +3.63D
    e. −6.67D

9) A patients' prescription is −13.00+2.00x067 at a vertex distance of 17 mm. If a frame were selected with a vertex distance of 22 mm, what lens power would have to be used?

    a. −10.42+1.79x067
    b. −12.90+2.48x067
    c. −10.51+1.98x067
    d. −13.90+2.26x067
    e. −12.21+1.67x067

10) An aphake is wearing +18 D glasses OU. He says that he sees better if he slides his glasses 2-mm down his nose. How is he changing his prescription?

    a. He is making his glasses stronger
    b. He is making his glasses weaker.
    c. He is adding base in prism to his glasses.
    d. He is adding base out prism to his glasses.
    e. He is creating a telescopic effect with his glasses.

11) A myope is wearing −10D glasses OU. She says that she sees better if she pushes her glasses closer to her eyes. How is she changing her prescription?

    a. She is making her glasses stronger
    b. She is making her glasses weaker.
    c. She is adding base in prism to her glasses.
    d. She is adding base out prism to her glasses.
    e. She is creating a telescopic effect with her glasses.

Subject: Index of refraction - Formula: U=n/u where U is in diopters, n is the index of refraction, and u is in meters.

12) Light is traveling from left to right in a liquid n=1.5. Light converges 10 cm to the right of a reference point. What is the vergence of light in the liquid?

    a. +5.00D
    b. +10.00D
    c. +15.00D
    d. −10.00D
    e. −5.00D

Subject: Prentice's rule - PD = hF where h is in cm and F is in diopters

13) A patient comes in wearing glasses +2D OD, –2D OS, complaining of vertical diplopia while reading. Both eyes are reading 5 mm down from the optical center. How much slab-off do you prescribe?
   a. 2 PD BU OD
   b. 4 PD BD OD
   c. 2 PD BU OS
   d. 4 PD BU OS
   e. No slab off prism is needed

14) A patient comes in wearing glasses +2D OD, +6D OS, complaining of vertical diplopia while reading. Both eyes are reading 8 mm down from the optical center. How much slab-off do you prescribe?
   a. 3.2 PD BU OD
   b. 3. 2PD BD OD
   c. 3. 2PD BU OS
   d. 3. 2 PD BD OS
   e. No slab off prism is needed

15) A patient comes in wearing glasses –3D OD, –8 D OS, complaining of vertical diplopia while reading. Both eyes are reading 7 mm down from the optical center. How much slab-off do you prescribe?
   a. 3.5 PD BU OD
   b. 7.7 PD BD OD
   c. 3.5 PD BD OS
   d. 3. 5 PD BU OS
   e. No slab off is needed

Subject: Lens Clock - Formula: $F_{true} = F_{lens\ clock}\ ((n'_{true} - n)/(n'_{lens\ clock} - n))$

16) Lens clock assumes that n is air and n' = 1.53 (crown glass)

A lens clock measures the power of a high index plastic surface (n=1.66) to be –5D. The lens clock has:
  a. Overestimated the power of the surface
  b. Underestimated the power of the surface
  c. Measured the power of the lens surface correctly
  d. Cannot be used to measure the power of high index plastic lenses
  e. None of the above

17) A patient with an RX of –3.00+2.50x180 OU wants to buy a pair of over the counter swimming goggles and he wants to know what power to buy. What do you recommend?
  a. –3.00D
  b. Plano sphere
  c. –1.75D
  d. –0.50D
  e. Power cannot be determined

18) A patient has never worn glasses before. You determine his prescription to be –4.00+6.00x 090. You decide to prescribe half of the actual cylinder in his prescription. In order to keep the same spherical equivalent as his actual prescription, you should prescribe:
  a. –1.00+3.00x090
  b. –2.50+3.00x090
  c. –4.00+3.00x090
  d. –2.00+3.00x090
  e. –3.00+3.00x090

19) A patient brings in a prescription of +5.75–3.25x063. Convert this to plus cylinder.
  a. +5.75+3.25x063
  b. +3.25+3.25x153
  c. +2.50+3.25x153
  d. +5.75+2.50x063
  e. +3.25+2.50x153

20) A patient brings in a prescription of –4.50+2.75x077. Convert this to minus cylinder.
    a. –4.50–2.75x077
    b. –1.75–2.75x077
    c. –2.75–2.75x167
    d. –1.75–2.75x167
    e. –2.75–2.75x077

21) Three optic points are located 33 cm, 25 cm, and 20 cm in front of a lens of +4.00 diopters; where are the three image points?
    a. +14.29cm, –12.5cm, +11.11cm
    b. +14.29cm, infinity, –11.11cm
    c. +100cm, infinity, –1.00cm
    d. –14.29cm, +12.5cm, +11.11cm
    e. –14.29cm, +12.5cm, –11.11cm

22) Three object points are located 100 cm, 50 cm, and 25 cm in front of a –2.00 diopter lens, where are the three image points?
    a. –33.33cm, –25cm, –16.67cm
    b. +33.33cm, +25cm, +16.67cm
    c. +100cm, infinity, –33.33cm
    d. +100cm, infinity, +33.33cm
    e. +100cm, infinity, +16.67cm

23) How much must an eye accommodate for a fixation point 10 cm in front of the eye?
    a. 10.00D
    b. 5.00D
    c. 2.50D
    d. 2.00D
    e. 3.00D

24) How much must a normal eye accommodate for a fixation point 20 cm in front of the eye?

    a. 10.00D

    b. 5.00D

    c. 2.50D

    d. 2.00D

    e. 3.00D

25) How much must a normal eye accommodate for a fixation point 33.3 cm in front of the eye?

    a. 10.00D

    b. 5.00D

    c. 2.50D

    d. 2.00D

    e. 3.00D

26) How much must a normal eye accommodate for a fixation point 50 cm in front of the eye?

    a. 10.00D

    b. 5.00D

    c. 2.50D

    d. 2.00D

    e. 3.00D

27) How much must an uncorrected 3.00D hyperope accommodate when viewing an object at 25cm?

    a. 1.00D

    b. 7.00D

    c. 4.00D

    d. 3.00D

    e. 9.25D

28) How much must an uncorrected 2.00D myope accommodate when viewing an object at 40cm?

    a.   2.00D
    b.   4.50D
    c.   0.50D
    d.   2.50D
    e.   1.00D

29) An object is located 33 cm in front of a +5.00 diopter lens; an eye located closely behind the lens can see the image distinctly without accommodation. What is the ametropia of this eye?

    a.   +8.00D
    b.   −8.00D
    c.   +2.00D
    d.   −2.00D
    e.   +5.00D

30) Three emmetropic eyes have amplitudes of accommodation of 5, 8, and 10 diopters respectively, what are their near points?

    a.   +20cm, +12.5cm, +10cm
    b.   −20cm, −12.5cm, −10cm
    c.   +8cm, +5cm, +4cm
    d.   −8cm, −5cm, −4cm
    e.   Cannot be calculated

31) The far point of an eye is found at 50 cm in front of the eye, the near point at 10 cm. What is the ametropia of this eye? What is its amplitude of accommodation?

    a.   −2.00, 8.00D
    b.   −2.00, 10.00D
    c.   −2.00, 12.00D
    d.   −10.00, 8.00D
    e.   −10.00, 12.00D

32) The far points of 4 eyes are found at 1 meter behind the cornea, 25 cm behind the cornea, 66.6 cm in front of the cornea, 20 cm in front of the cornea. What are the powers of the correcting lenses placed at the cornea?

    a.   −1.00D, −4.00D, +1.50D, +5.00D
    b.   +1.00D, +6.25D, −1.66D, −2.00D
    c.   +1.00D, +4.00D, −1.50D, −5.00D
    d.   −1.00D, −6.25D, +1.66D, +2.00D
    e.   −1.00D, −4.00D, +1.66D, +5.00D

33) Assume an amplitude of accommodation of 5.00 diopters in all cases noted on Problem 32, what are the respective near points?

    a.   16.67cm, 11.11cm, 28.75cm, infinity
    b.   25cm, 80cm, 15cm, 14.29cm
    c.   25cm, 100cm, 15.39cm, 10cm
    d.   16.67cm, 8.89cm, 29.94cm, 33cm
    e.   16.67cm, 11.11cm, 29.94, infinity

34) Calculate the magnification of a +28 D hand-held magnifier if the object is held at f:

    a.   11.2x
    b.   7.0x
    c.   4.2x
    d.   2.8x
    e.   None of the above

35) When dealing with multiple lens systems, the total magnification is:

    a.   The sum of each component magnifier
    b.   The average of all the component magnifiers
    c.   The product of each component magnifier
    d.   The product of each component magnifier divided by the number of component magnifiers used
    e.   None of the above

36) What is the accommodation required through a 3x Galilean telescope if the object is 25 cm away?

    a.   48D
    b.   12D
    c.   24D
    d.   36D
    e.   None of the above

37) What power reading cap is needed for a Galilean telescope used to view an object at 10cm?

    a.   4.00D
    b.   5.00D
    c.   2.00D
    d.   1.00D
    e.   None of the above

38) What power reading cap is needed for a Galilean telescope used to view an object at 25cm?

    a.   4.00D
    b.   5.00D
    c.   2.00D
    d.   1.00D
    e.   None of the above

39) What power reading cap is needed for a Galilean telescope used to view an object at 50cm?

    a.   4.00D
    b.   5.00D
    c.   2.00D
    d.   1.00D
    e.   None of the above

40) What power reading cap is needed for a Galilean telescope used to view an object at 100cm?

    a. 4.00D

    b. 5.00D

    c. 2.00D

    d. 1.00D

    e. None of the above

41) +6D and –15D lenses are used to make a Galilean telescope. Which of the following statements is true for an object at 5 cm?

    a. The image is real and to the right of the objective lens.

    b. Total magnification is 1%

    c. The image of a near object is coincident with that for far.

    d. The image is inside the telescope.

    e. None of the above.

42) +6D and –15D lenses are used to make a Galilean telescope. Which of the following statements is true for an object at infinity?

    a. The image is inverted and to the right of the objective lens.

    b. Total magnification is 2.5x.

    c. The image of a near object is coincident with that for far.

    d. The image is inside the telescope.

    e. None of the above.

43) +6 D and +15 D lenses are used to make a Keplerian telescope. Which of the following statements is true for an object at infinity?

    a. The image is erect and to the right of the objective lens.

    b. Total magnification is 15%

    c. The image of a near object is coincident with that for far.

    d. The image is inside the telescope.

    e. None of the above.

44) What is the tube length of a telescope fabricated with a +4D and a -20D lens, focused at infinity?

    a.   20cm
    b.   25 cm
    c.   15cm
    d.   10cm
    e.   None of the above

45) What is the tube length of a telescope fabricated with a +5D and a +20D lens, focused at infinity?

    a.   20cm
    b.   25cm
    c.   15cm
    d.   10cm
    e.   None of the above

46) What is the magnification of the telescope fabricated with a +5D and a +20D lens?

    a.   2x
    b.   3x
    c.   4x
    d.   5x
    e.   6x

47) If we increase the reference distance for simple magnifiers from 25 to 50 cm, what will happen to the effective image size?

    a.   It appears 2x larger
    b.   No change would occur
    c.   It appears smaller by half
    d.   It appears 3x larger
    e.   It appears smaller by one third

48) Consider a concave lens of –15 D. If the object distance is 20 cm behind the lens, describe the image nature and position:
    a.   The image is virtual and located 10 cm in front of the lens.
    b.   The image is virtual and located 5 cm in front of the lens.
    c.   The image is real and located 10 cm behind the lens.
    d.   The image is virtual and located 20 cm in front of the lens.
    e.   The image is real and located 5 cm behind the lens.

49) How far away from a plane mirror is the image of an object of vergence +5 D?
    a.   2 m
    b.   2 cm
    c.   5 cm
    d.   5 mm
    e.   None of the above

50) An object is 40 cm in front of a refracting surface of power +10 D. Which of the following is incorrect?
    a.   The object vergence is –2.5 D
    b.   The image is 13.3 cm to the right of the lens
    c.   The image is real
    d.   The image vergence is –7.5 D
    e.   The image is inverted

Answers:

You can take practice exams online at:

http://www.medrounds.org/ophthalmology-board-review/exam/

1. .... d

2. .... a

3. c

Light converges to 50cm to the right of the lens. This is the reference point for the vergence of light. At 15cm to the right of the lens, light is now 35cm from the convergent point. Vergence is $= 100/u = 100/35 = +2.86D$. This is positive because light is converging to the reference point.

4. .... d

Light converges to 50cm to the right of the lens. This is the reference point for the vergence of light. At 40cm to the right of the lens, light is now 10cm from the convergent point. Vergence is $= 100/u = 100/10 = +10D$. This is positive because light is converging to the reference point.

5. .... d

Light converges to 50cm to the right of the lens. This is the reference point for the vergence of light. At 55cm to the right of the lens, light is now 5cm from the convergent point and diverging. Divergence is $= (-) 100/u = (-) 100/5 = -20D$. This is negative because light is diverging from the reference point.

6. .... b

Light converges to 50cm to the right of the lens. This is the reference point for the vergence of light. At 150cm to the right of the lens, light is now 100cm from the convergent point and diverging. Divergence is $= (-) 100/u = (-) 100/100 = -1D$. This is negative because light is diverging from the reference point.

7......... b

> Light converges to 16.67cm to the right of the lens (vergence of +6D). This is the reference point for the vergence of light. After travel of 10mm in air, light has traveled 1cm or within 15.67cm of the convergent point. Vergence is = 100/u = 100/15.67 = +6.38D. This is positive because light is converging to the reference point.

8......... b

> Light diverges to 12.50cm to the right of the lens (divergence of –8D). This is the reference point for the divergence of light. After travel of 15mm in air, light has traveled 14cm from the lens. Divergence is = (–)100/u = (–)100/14 = –7.14D. This is negative because light is diverging from the lens.

9......... d

> To solve this problem, convert the prescription into a powercross consisting of –13.00D at 67 degrees and –11.00D at 157 degrees. Apply the lens effectivity formula. With increased vertex distance, the minus lenses need to be more minus; thus, the new powercross will be –13.90D at 67 degrees and –11.64D at 157 degrees. The prescription is –13.90+2.26x067.

10........ a

11........ a

12........ c

> Use index of refraction formula: U=n/u where U is in diopters, n is the index of refraction, and u is in meters.

13........ c

> 2 Prism Diopters Base Up OS. Looking 5 mm down from the optical center produces 1 PD BU OD and 1 PD BD OS with an effective prism power of 2 PD BD OS. 2 PD BU OS will neutralize this. Slab-off is prescribed for the most minus or least plus lens.

14. .... a

> 3.2 Prism Diopters Base Up OD. At 8 mm down from the optical center, there is 1.6 PD BU OD and 4.8 PD BU OS with a total 3.2 PD BU effect OS. Slab-off is prescribed in the most minus or least plus lens; thus, 3.2 PD BU OD is needed to neutralize the prismatic effect.

15. .... d

> 3.5 Prism Diopters base up OS. At 7 mm down from the optical center, there is 2.1 PD BD OD and 5.6 PD BD OS with a total of 3.5 PD BD OS. Slab-off is prescribed for the most minus or least plus lens; thus, 3.5 PD BU OS is needed to neutralize the prismatic effect.

16. .... b

17. c

> The spherical equivalent of $-3.00+2.50 \times 180$ is $-1.75D$. To calculate the spherical equivalent, take 1/2 of the cylinder power and combine it with the sphere power. While wearing goggles, the patient will not need cylinder so an RX of $-1.75D$ is needed.

18. .... b

To calculate the spherical equivalent, take 1/2 of the cylinder power and combine it with the sphere power. In this case, a decrease in $+3.00$ diopters of cylinder will result in a decrease of -1.50 in the sphere power to maintain a spherical equivalence of -1.00.

19. c

20. .... d

21. c

22. .... a

23. .... a

24. .... b

25. .... e

26......... d

27......... b

> The hyperope needs 4.00D of accommodation and also an extra 3.00D to overcome his refractive error.

28......... c

> The uncorrected myope can see well at 50cm, but needs 0.50D of accommodation to view an object at 40cm.

29......... c

> An eye without refractive error needs a +3.00D lens to see an object at 33cm without accommodation. A +2.00D hyperope requires a +5.00D lens to see an image at 33cm without accommodation.

30......... a

31......... a

32......... c

33......... c

34......... b

35......... c

36......... d

> 36D where the approximate accommodation required is given by $A_{oc} = M^2U$, where A_{oc} = vergence at the eyepiece = accommodation, U = object vergence at the objective = 1/u, M = the magnification of the telescope.

37......... e

38......... a

39......... c

40......... d

41......... d

42......... b

43......... e

44......... a

45......... b

46......... c

47......... a

48......... a

49......... e

50......... d

Bibliography

1. Duke-Elder WS. The adjustment of the optical system: Accommodation. In: WS Duke-Elder, *Text-book of ophthalmology. Volume 1. The Development, Form and Function of the Visual Apparatus*. St. Louis: C. V. Mosby, Co.; 1938; p. 752-65.

2. Duke-Elder WS, Abrams D. Chapter XIII. Anisekonia. In: WS Duke-Elder, editor, *System of Ophthalmology. Volume V. Ophthalmic Optics and Refraction*. St. Louis: C. V. Mosby, Co.; 1963 (1970); p. 513-34.

3. Appleton B. *Clinical Optics* (Ophthalmic Technical Skills Series, vol. 2). Thorofare, NJ: Slack, Inc.; 1990.

4. Optics*, Refraction, and Contacts Lenses* (Basic and Clinical Science Course, 1998-1999). San Francisco, CA: American Academy of Ophthalmology; 1998.

5. MacInnis BJ. *Ophthalmology Board Review of Optics and Refraction*. St. Louis: Mosby; 1993.

6. Refraction and Clinical Optics. Chapters 31-52, 58, 60. In: W Tasman; E Jaeger, editors, *Duane's Clinical Ophthalmology. Vol. 1*. Philadelphia: Lippincott Williams & Wilkins; 2005.

7. *Section 3. Optics, Refraction, and Contacts Lenses* (Basic and Clinical Science Course, 2004-2005). San Francisco, CA: American Academy of Ophthalmology; 2004.

Index

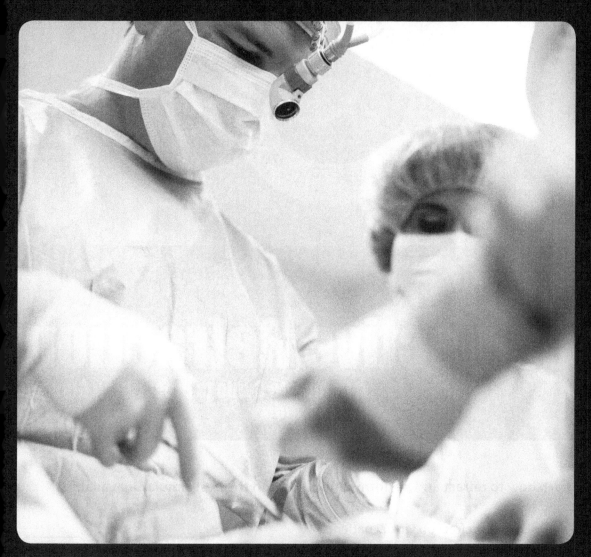

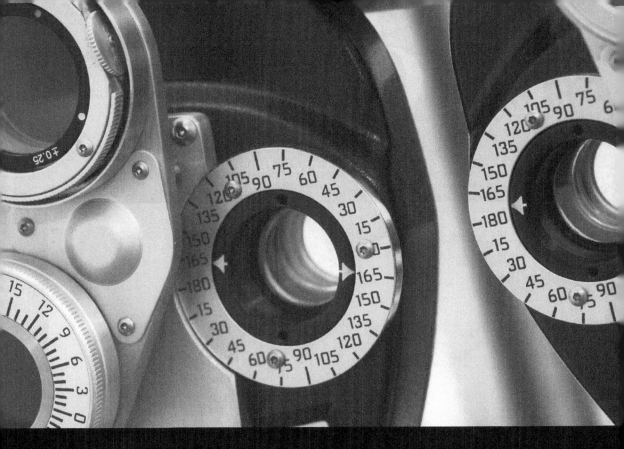

Introduction to

Subjective Refraction

A Complete Guide to Prescribing Glasses

Learn how to refract and perform retinoscopy on the best simulator available.

- Learn to refract on virtual patients.
- Sharpen your skills with clinical scenarios.
- Practice with PLUS or MINUS cylinder phoropter.
- Refine your retinoscopy skills.
- This is the best virtual simulator available.
- Lessons are animated in FLASH.
- Outstanding educational tool to teach the basics of prescribing glasses to students, technicians, and residents.

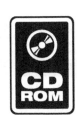

CD ROM

www.medrounds.org/refract/

CPSIA information can be obtained at www.ICGtesting.com
Printed in the USA
LVOW02s0314130214

373382LV00004B/141/P